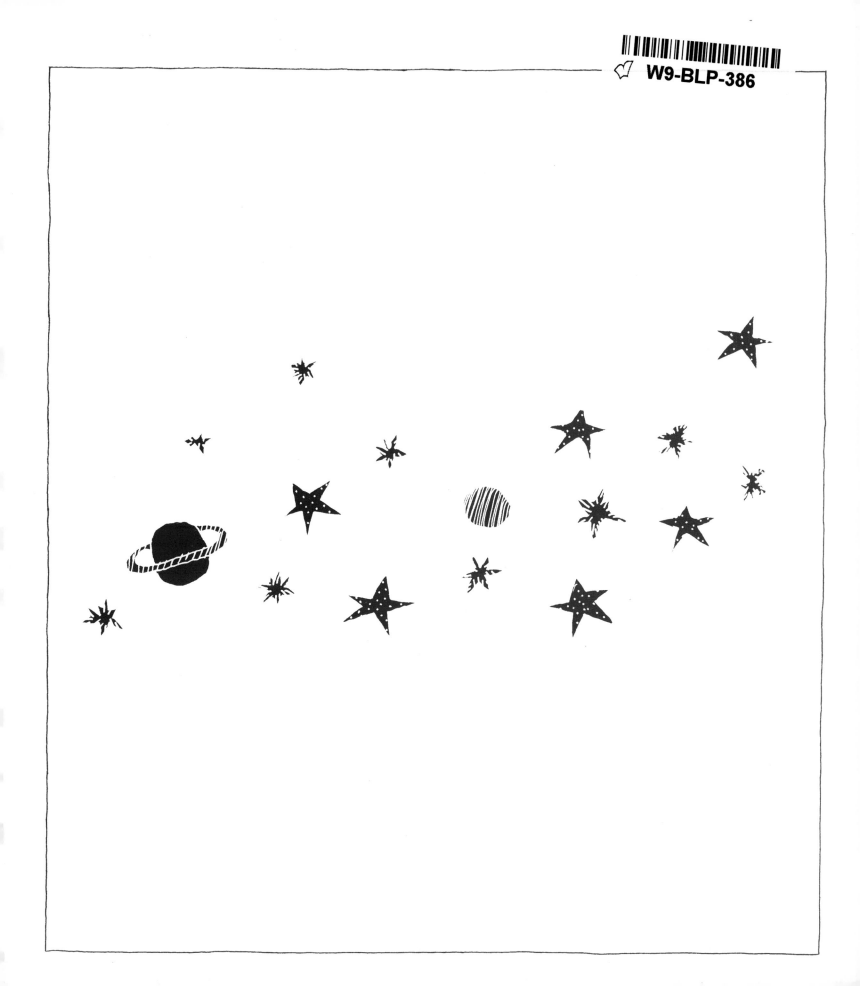

Tangles

Sarah Leavitt

A story about Alzheimer's, my mother, and me

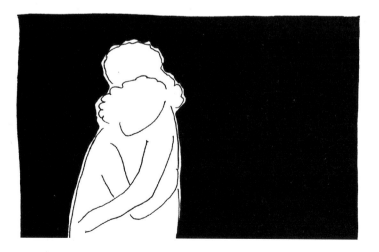

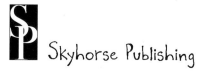 Skyhorse Publishing

Copyright © 2012 Sarah Leavitt

Skyhorse Publishing books may be purchased in bulk at special discounts for sales promotion, corporate gifts, fund-raising, or educational purposes. Special editions can also be created to specifications. For details, contact the Special Sales Department, Skyhorse Publishing, 307 West 36th Street, 11th Floor, New York, NY 10018 or info@skyhorsepublishing.com.

Visit our website at www.skyhorsepublishing.com.

10 9 8 7 6 5 4 3 2 1

Library of Congress Cataloging-in-Publication Data is available on file.
ISBN: 978-1-61608-639-8

First published in Canada by Freehand Books

Edited by Robyn Read
Art direction by Natalie Olsen, www.kisscutdesign.com
Author photo by Teri Snelgrove

Excerpt from "the Cambridge ladies who live in furnished souls," in Complete Poems: 1904–1962. Edited by George J. Firmage. Copyright 1923, 1951, 1991 by The Trustees of the E.E. Cummings Trust. Copyright 1976 by George James Firmage. Reprinted by permission of Liveright Publishing Corporation/WW Norton + Company, Inc.

Printed in China

For my father Robert and my sister Hannah.

For my dearest companion Donimo and my drawing friend Mary,
because I would never have finished this without you.

Most of all, for my mother Midge, whom I will miss forever.

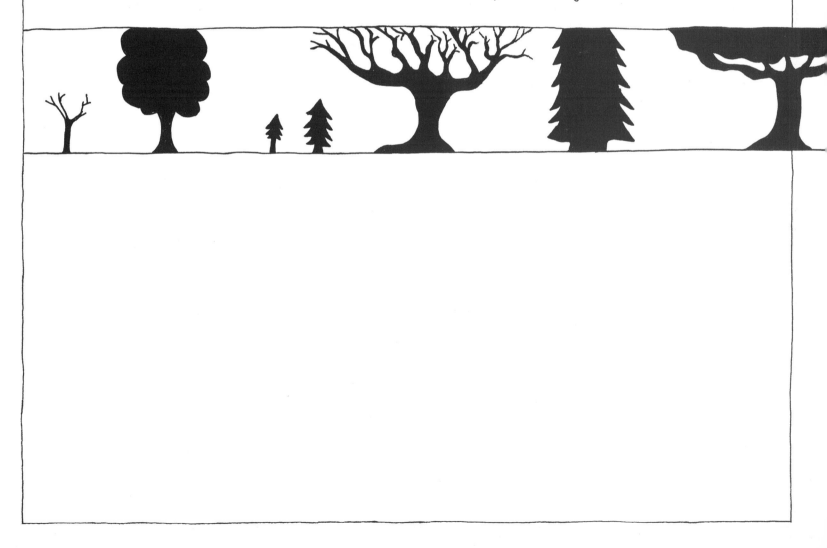

Introduction

I've always had a really bad memory. So when my mother got Alzheimer's disease, I knew that I had to record what was happening to her and to our family. I wanted to be able to look back over my notes and remember all the moments of craziness, beauty, and tragedy—and not lose any of them.

Mom started showing symptoms of Alzheimer's in 1996, when she was only 52. Our family ran through all the possible explanations—job loss, depression, menopause—until finally we realized it must be something neurological. She was diagnosed with Alzheimer's in 1998. For the next six years my father cared for her, eventually with the help of hired caregivers. Mom's sisters, Debbie and Sukey, and my sister Hannah and I helped as much as we could.

I lived in Vancouver and my parents lived in Fredericton, New Brunswick. I visited two or three times a year, and took notes and drew pictures the whole time I was there.

I often felt like Harriet the Spy, or, in darker moments, like a vulture hovering and waiting for Mom to say or do something that I could record and preserve, even as she slipped away from me. Sometimes she would pull on the page or grab my pen as I tried to write. The pen would skid and make a mark and I'd label the mark: "Mom moved my pen." I wanted to keep every trace of her.

I ended up with a box of notes and sketches, some careful and considered, some dashed off in the middle of a crisis and barely legible or blotched with dried tears. There are small notes I made on scraps of paper right as things were happening, like at the dinner table when Mom started talking to the broccoli.

During Mom's illness, I started using some of my notes to write stories and essays about what was happening. I imagined writing a book. About nine months after Mom died I went through the journals, sketchbooks, and scraps of paper I'd collected over the six years of her illness. I chose a small number of drawings and notes, compiled them into a booklet, and made a few colour copies. I realized that instead of writing prose about my mother I wanted to do a graphic memoir, and I spent the next four years writing and drawing this book.

My mother loved her family with a fierce and absolute love. Alzheimer's disease tore her away from us and from herself in a cruel, relentless progression of losses. But even as she lost her ability to form sentences, and stopped saying our names, and stopped understanding ideas like sister, daughter, or husband, she would still cry out with joy when we came into the room.

I created this book to remember her as she was before she got sick, but also to remember her as she was during her illness, the ways in which she was transformed and the ways in which parts of her endured. As my mother changed, I changed too, forced to reconsider my own identity as a daughter and as an adult and to recreate my relationship with my mother.

This is the story that I have pieced together from my memories, my notes, and my sketches. Other people in my family may remember things differently. In the end, this is only my story: the tangled story of my mother, and me, and Alzheimer's.

Sarah Leavitt
Vancouver
March 2010

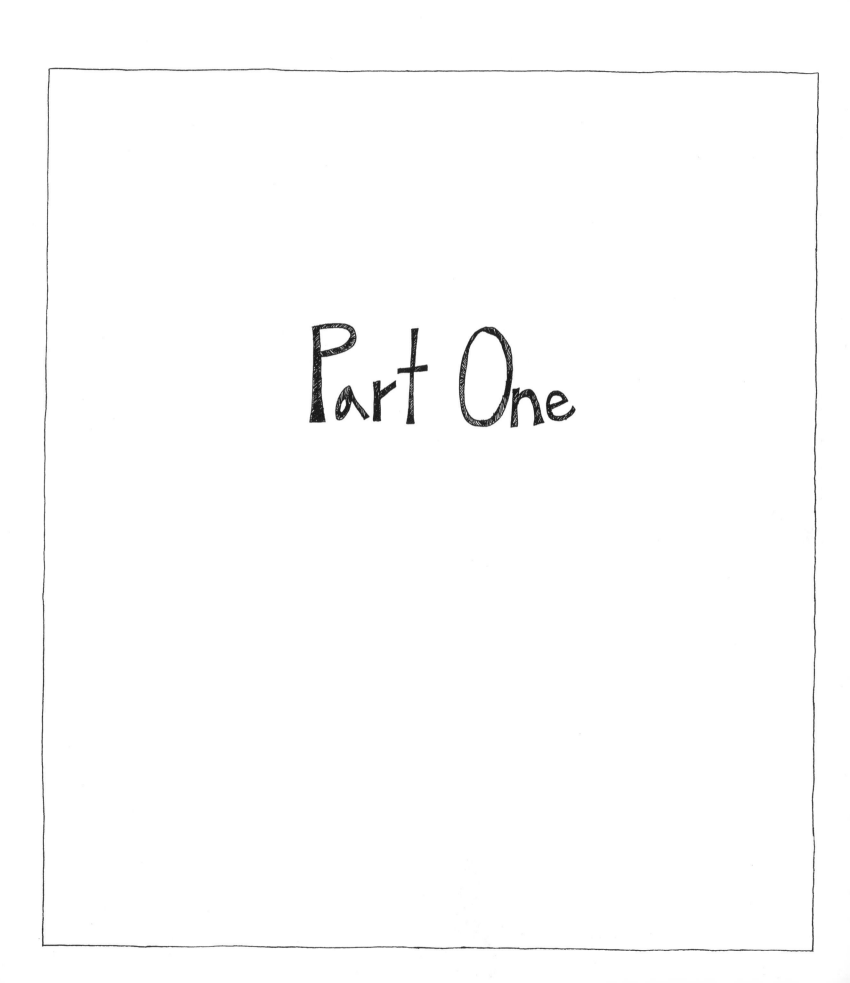

Part One

Nightmares

When I was little, we lived in the country in an old rented farmhouse. I slept upstairs at the back of the house in a creaky bed that the owners had left behind. The flowers in the wallpaper changed shape at night. Rats and squirrels ran up and down inside the walls.

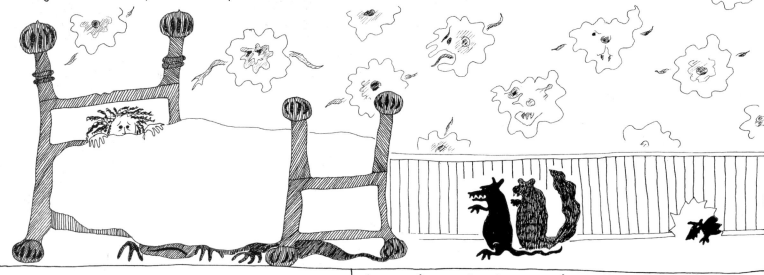

Evil creatures lurked under the bed, so I couldn't get out unless I kind of jumped away from the bed.

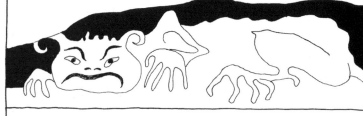

I never forgot the chapter in Little House on the Prairie where a mouse chews off some of Pa's hair. I buried myself under the covers until I fell asleep.

But then the nightmares started. A robber caught me. Or a Black Rider. Or a Flying Monkey.

Aaaah!

I'd wake myself up screaming.

MOM!?!

And then I'd wait...

MOM

to be rescued.

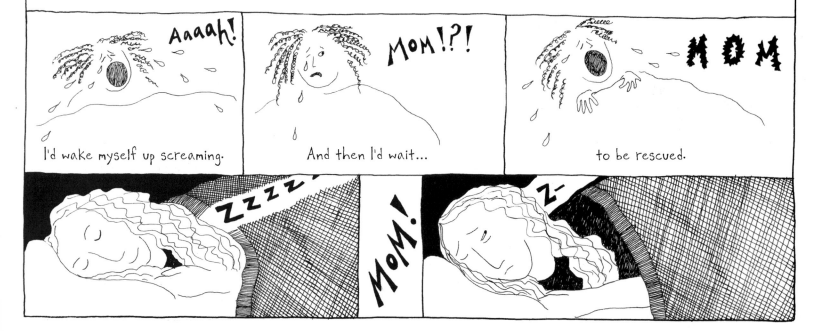

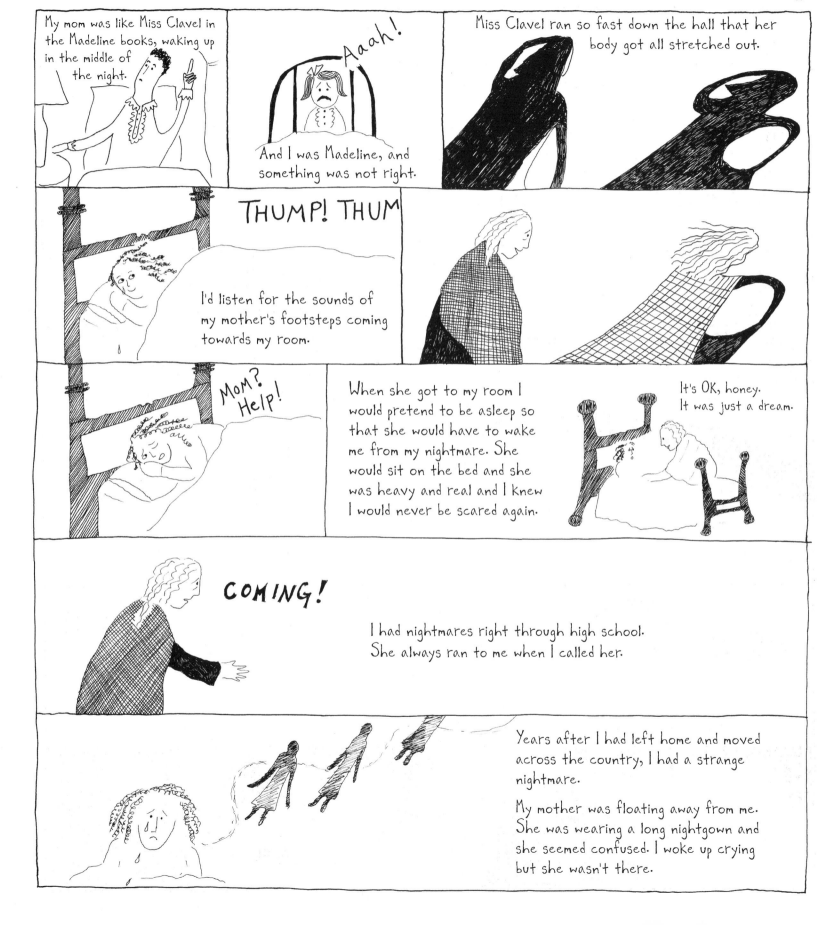

Sisters

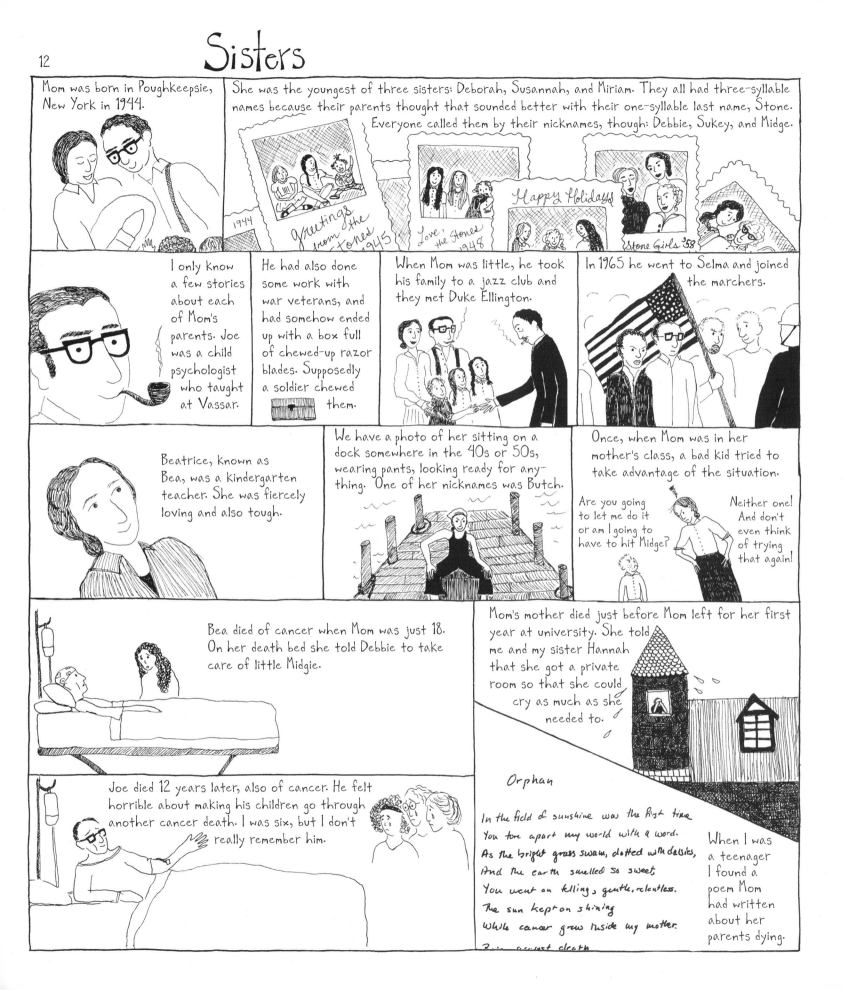

Mom was born in Poughkeepsie, New York in 1944.

She was the youngest of three sisters: Deborah, Susannah, and Miriam. They all had three-syllable names because their parents thought that sounded better with their one-syllable last name, Stone. Everyone called them by their nicknames, though: Debbie, Sukey, and Midge.

1944

Greetings from the Stones 1945

Love, the Stones 1948

Happy Holidays

Stone Girls '58

I only know a few stories about each of Mom's parents. Joe was a child psychologist who taught at Vassar.

He had also done some work with war veterans, and had somehow ended up with a box full of chewed-up razor blades. Supposedly a soldier chewed them.

When Mom was little, he took his family to a jazz club and they met Duke Ellington.

In 1965 he went to Selma and joined the marchers.

Beatrice, known as Bea, was a kindergarten teacher. She was fiercely loving and also tough.

We have a photo of her sitting on a dock somewhere in the 40s or 50s, wearing pants, looking ready for anything. One of her nicknames was Butch.

Once, when Mom was in her mother's class, a bad kid tried to take advantage of the situation.

Are you going to let me do it or am I going to have to hit Midge?

Neither one! And don't even think of trying that again!

Bea died of cancer when Mom was just 18. On her death bed she told Debbie to take care of little Midgie.

Mom's mother died just before Mom left for her first year at university. She told me and my sister Hannah that she got a private room so that she could cry as much as she needed to.

Joe died 12 years later, also of cancer. He felt horrible about making his children go through another cancer death. I was six, but I don't really remember him.

Orphan

In the field of sunshine was the first time
You tore apart my world with a word.
As the bright grass swam, dotted with daisies,
And the earth smelled so sweet
You went on telling, gentle, relentless.
The sun kept on shining
While cancer grew inside my mother.

When I was a teenager I found a poem Mom had written about her parents dying.

No matter how much time went by, Debbie, Sukey, and Midge talked and cried about their parents as if they had just recently died.

Debbie moved to a small town not far from Poughkeepsie. She lived with her son in a tiny house.

Mom ended up in the country in Maine, and eventually moved to Canada.

Sukey moved to Philadelphia with her husband.

They were all teachers. Debbie taught at an alternative school.

Sukey taught preschool.

Mom taught kindergarten like her mother had.

The sisters saw each other often. They would kiss and hug and retreat into their own world, where they talked about their parents and sang for hours in three-part harmony: folk songs, children's songs, Christmas carols (they were Jewish but definitely not religious).

John Henry was a little baby Sittin' on his daddy's knee

But the banks are made of marble, with a guard at every door and the vaults are stuffed with silver

Children go where I send thee! How shall I send thee?

They all sounded exactly alike on the phone.

Hello, Sarah darling!

They were so close.

There was one story about one of them hitting another one with a hairbrush at some point when they were kids.

OW!

But that was the exception. The sisters never seemed to get mad at each other or even disagree.

One summer, when I was 13 and my sister Hannah was 11, Mom was at her wit's end.

We talked back all the time.

We left huge messes everywhere.

And we fought almost constantly.

YANK!

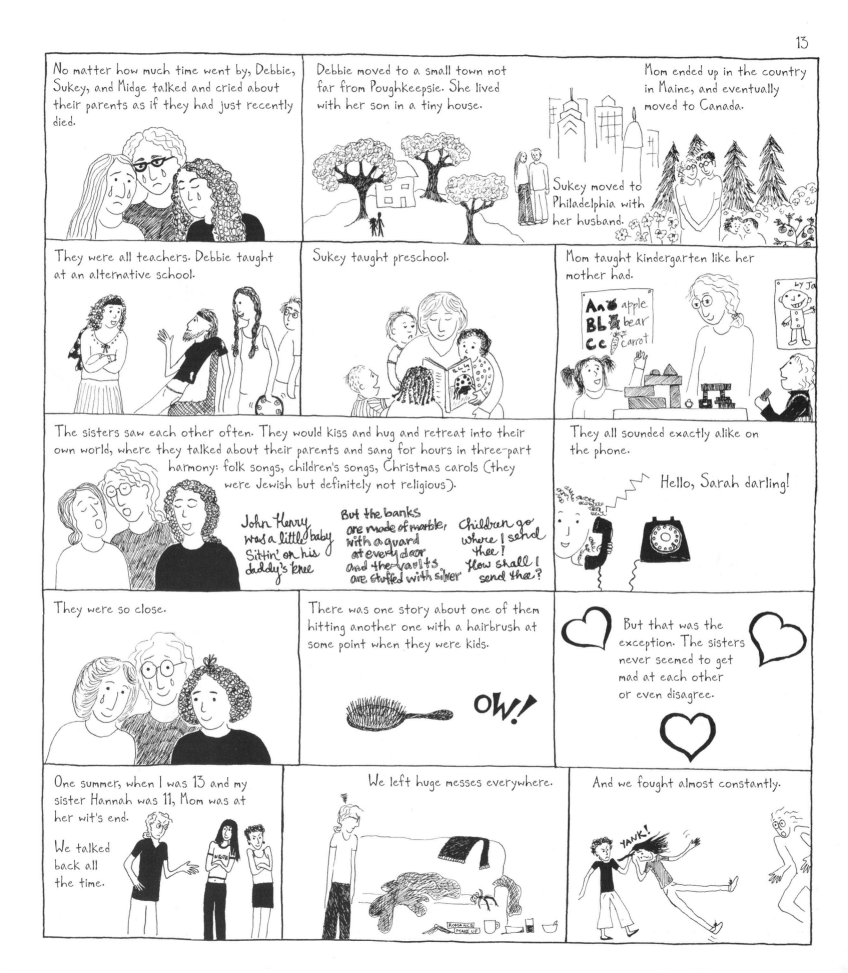

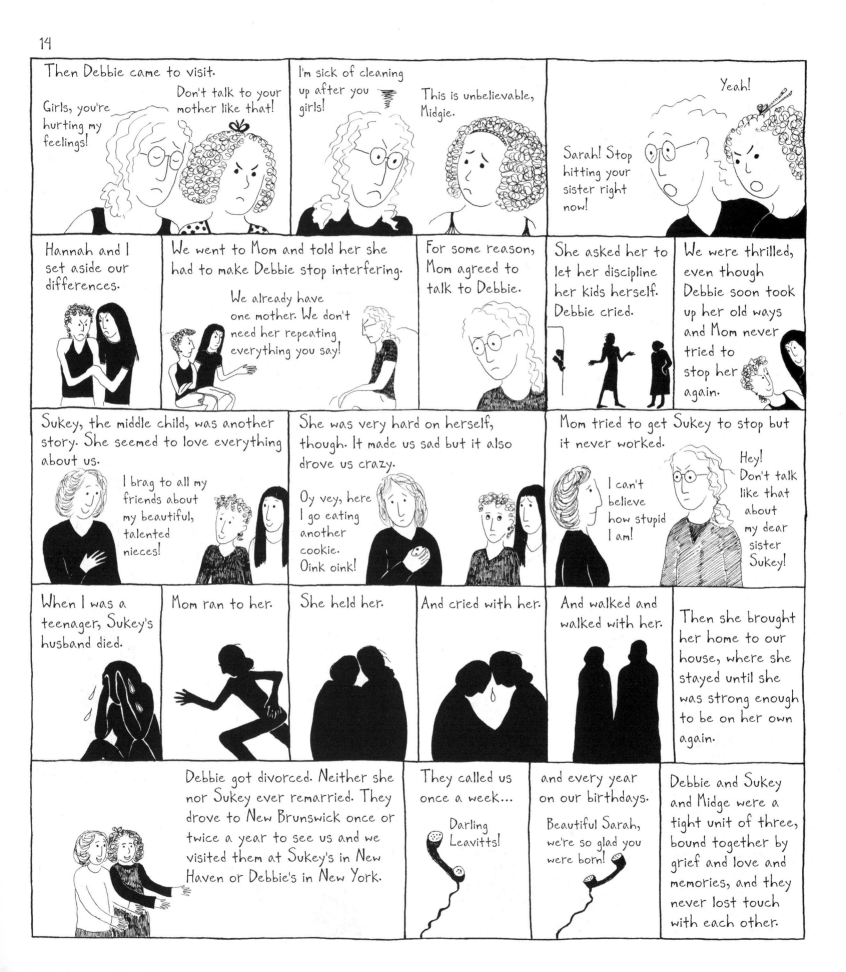

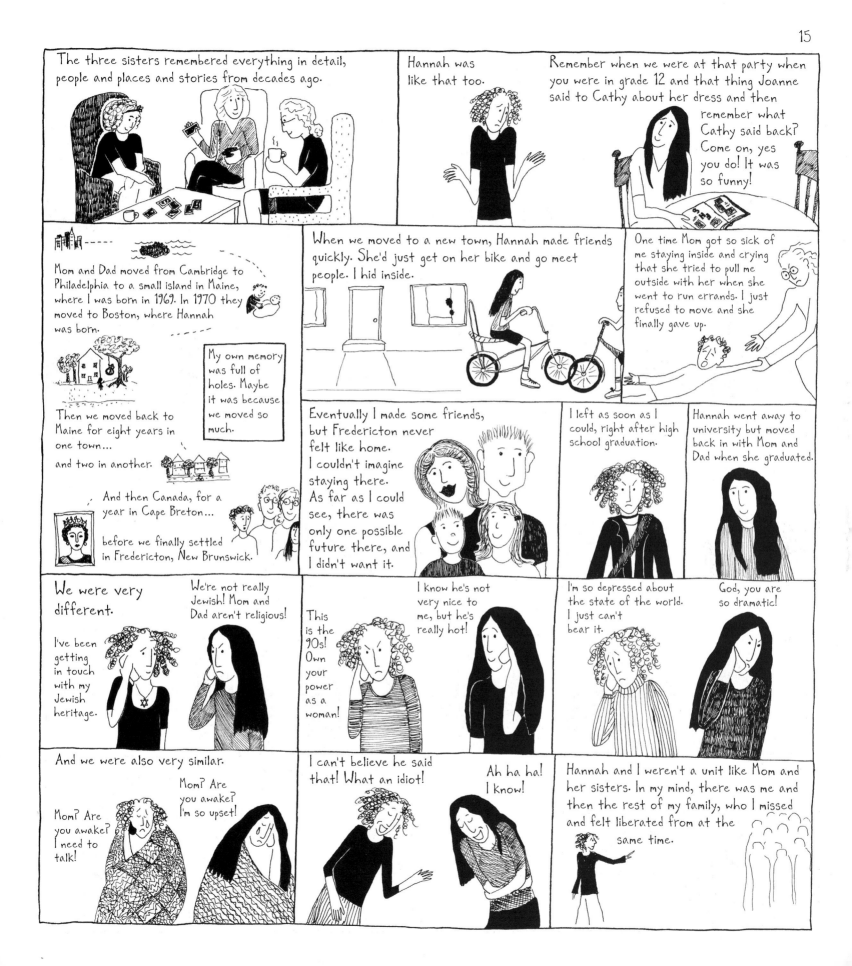

The three sisters remembered everything in detail, people and places and stories from decades ago.

Hannah was like that too.

Remember when we were at that party when you were in grade 12 and that thing Joanne said to Cathy about her dress and then remember what Cathy said back? Come on, yes you do! It was so funny!

Mom and Dad moved from Cambridge to Philadelphia to a small island in Maine, where I was born in 1969. In 1970 they moved to Boston, where Hannah was born.

My own memory was full of holes. Maybe it was because we moved so much.

When we moved to a new town, Hannah made friends quickly. She'd just get on her bike and go meet people. I hid inside.

One time Mom got so sick of me staying inside and crying that she tried to pull me outside with her when she went to run errands. I just refused to move and she finally gave up.

Then we moved back to Maine for eight years in one town...

and two in another.

And then Canada, for a year in Cape Breton...

before we finally settled in Fredericton, New Brunswick.

Eventually I made some friends, but Fredericton never felt like home. I couldn't imagine staying there. As far as I could see, there was only one possible future there, and I didn't want it.

I left as soon as I could, right after high school graduation.

Hannah went away to university but moved back in with Mom and Dad when she graduated.

We were very different.

I've been getting in touch with my Jewish heritage.

We're not really Jewish! Mom and Dad aren't religious!

This is the 90s! Own your power as a woman!

I know he's not very nice to me, but he's really hot!

I'm so depressed about the state of the world. I just can't bear it.

God, you are so dramatic!

And we were also very similar.

Mom? Are you awake? I need to talk!

Mom? Are you awake? I'm so upset!

I can't believe he said that! What an idiot!

Ah ha ha! I know!

Hannah and I weren't a unit like Mom and her sisters. In my mind, there was me and then the rest of my family, who I missed and felt liberated from at the same time.

Long Distance

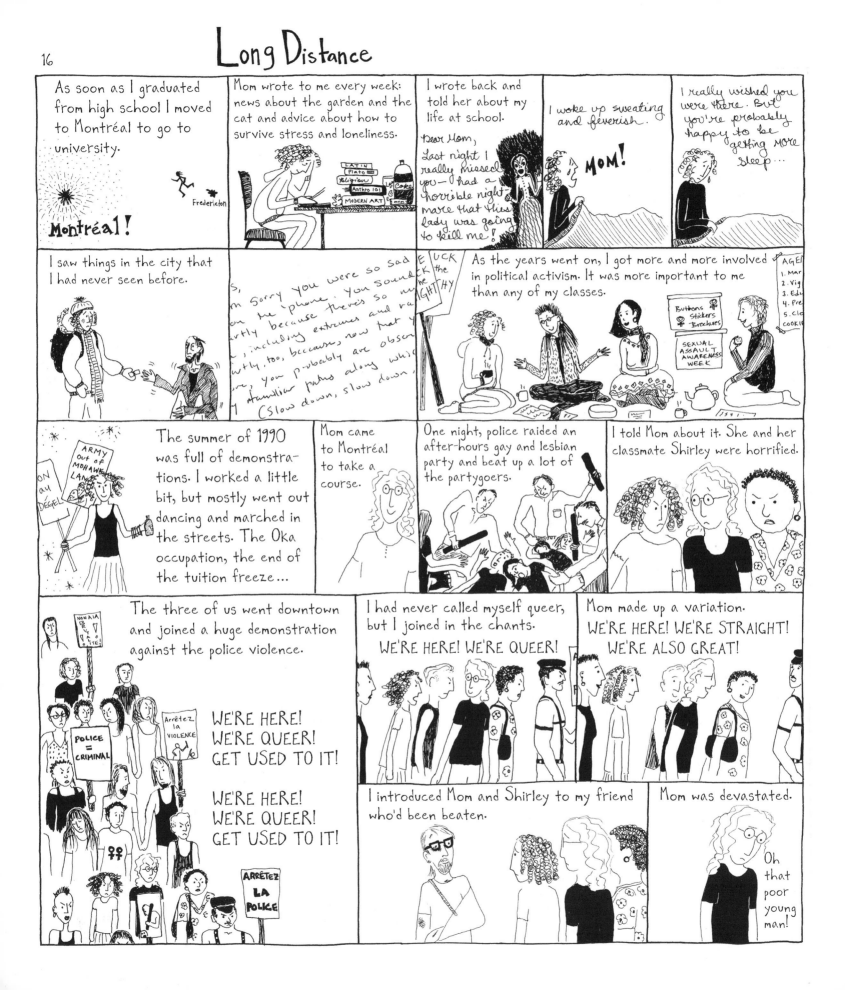

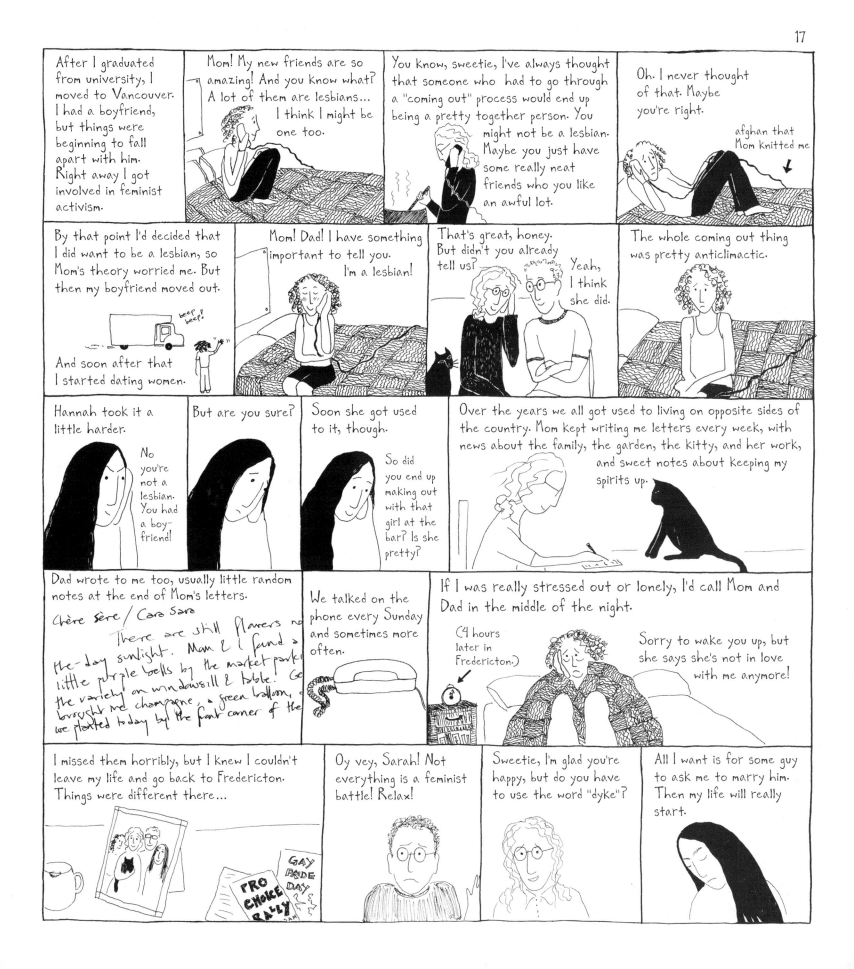

Signs

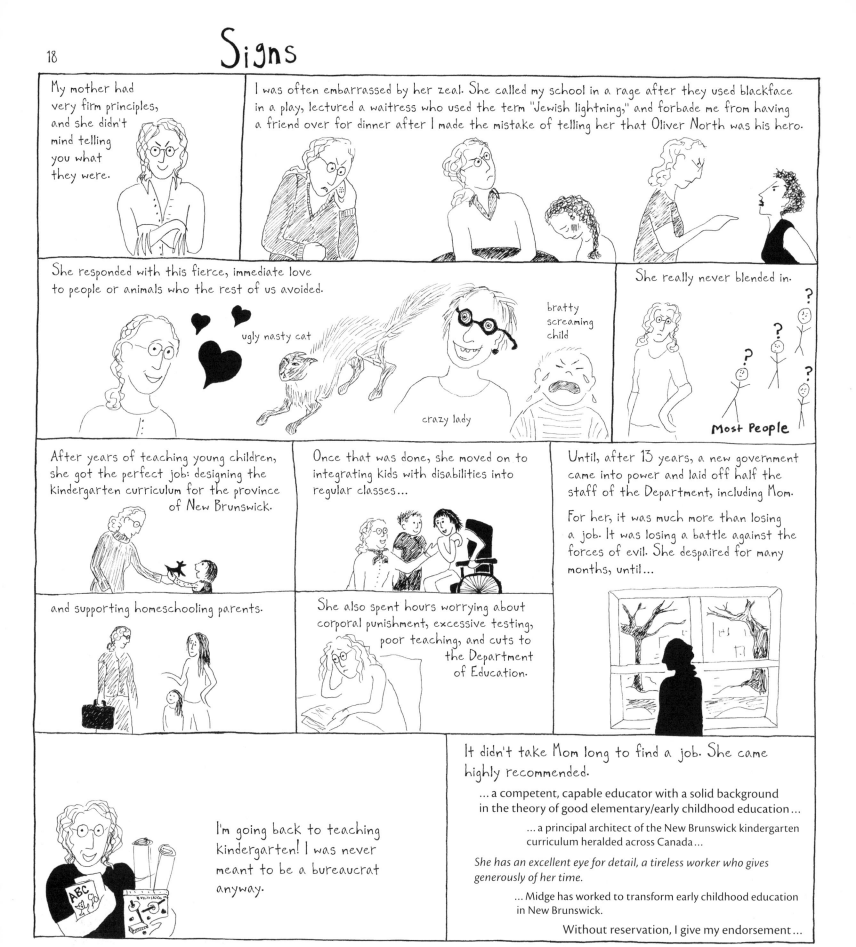

My mother had very firm principles, and she didn't mind telling you what they were.

I was often embarrassed by her zeal. She called my school in a rage after they used blackface in a play, lectured a waitress who used the term "Jewish lightning," and forbade me from having a friend over for dinner after I made the mistake of telling her that Oliver North was his hero.

She responded with this fierce, immediate love to people or animals who the rest of us avoided.

ugly nasty cat

bratty screaming child

crazy lady

She really never blended in.

? ? ? ?

Most People

After years of teaching young children, she got the perfect job: designing the kindergarten curriculum for the province of New Brunswick.

and supporting homeschooling parents.

Once that was done, she moved on to integrating kids with disabilities into regular classes...

She also spent hours worrying about corporal punishment, excessive testing, poor teaching, and cuts to the Department of Education.

Until, after 13 years, a new government came into power and laid off half the staff of the Department, including Mom.

For her, it was much more than losing a job. It was losing a battle against the forces of evil. She despaired for many months, until...

I'm going back to teaching kindergarten! I was never meant to be a bureaucrat anyway.

ABC

It didn't take Mom long to find a job. She came highly recommended.

... a competent, capable educator with a solid background in the theory of good elementary/early childhood education...

... a principal architect of the New Brunswick kindergarten curriculum heralded across Canada...

She has an excellent eye for detail, a tireless worker who gives generously of her time.

... Midge has worked to transform early childhood education in New Brunswick.

Without reservation, I give my endorsement...

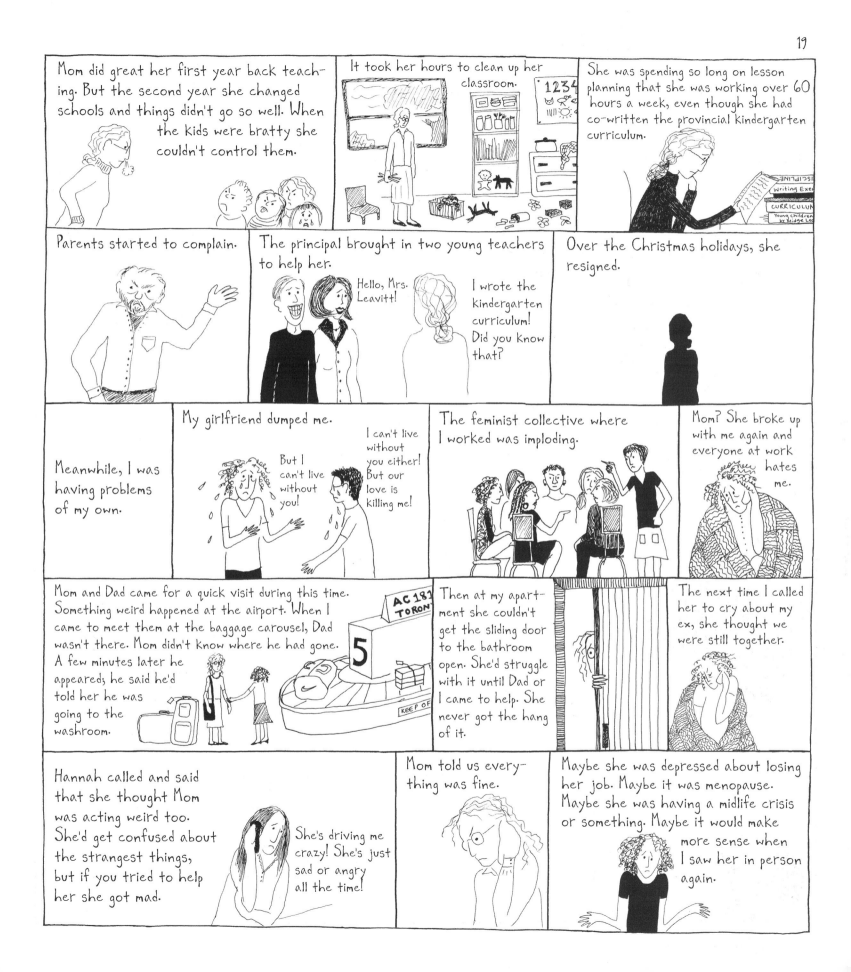

Arrival

In the summer of 1998 I went to Fredericton. It takes a whole day to travel there from Vancouver.

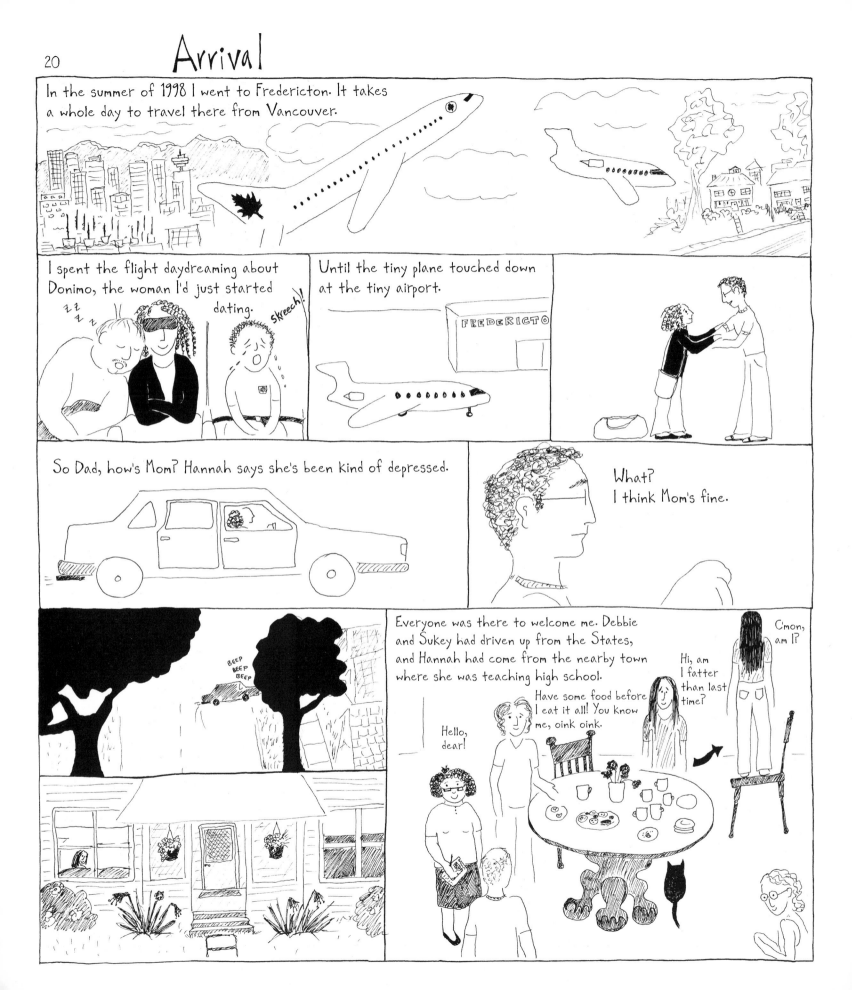

I spent the flight daydreaming about Donimo, the woman I'd just started dating.

Skreech!

Until the tiny plane touched down at the tiny airport.

FREDERICTO

So Dad, how's Mom? Hannah says she's been kind of depressed.

What? I think Mom's fine.

BEEP BEEP BEEP

Everyone was there to welcome me. Debbie and Sukey had driven up from the States, and Hannah had come from the nearby town where she was teaching high school.

Hello, dear!

Have some food before I eat it all! You know me, oink oink.

Hi, am I fatter than last time?

Cmon, am I?

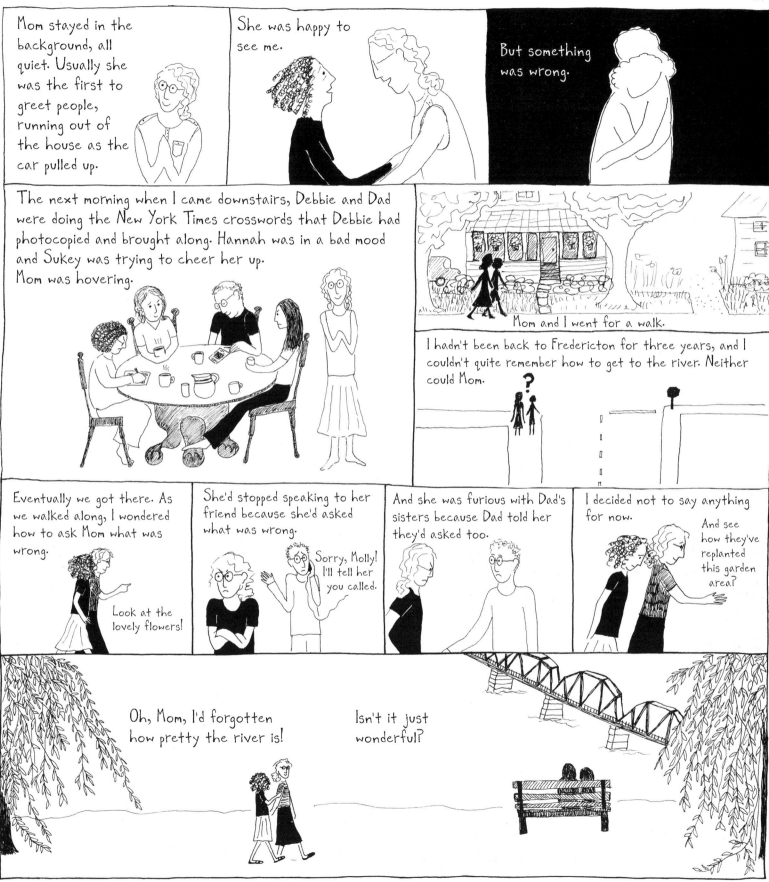

Mom stayed in the background, all quiet. Usually she was the first to greet people, running out of the house as the car pulled up.

She was happy to see me.

But something was wrong.

The next morning when I came downstairs, Debbie and Dad were doing the New York Times crosswords that Debbie had photocopied and brought along. Hannah was in a bad mood and Sukey was trying to cheer her up. Mom was hovering.

Mom and I went for a walk.

I hadn't been back to Fredericton for three years, and I couldn't quite remember how to get to the river. Neither could Mom.

Eventually we got there. As we walked along, I wondered how to ask Mom what was wrong.

Look at the lovely flowers!

She'd stopped speaking to her friend because she'd asked what was wrong.

Sorry, Molly! I'll tell her you called.

And she was furious with Dad's sisters because Dad told her they'd asked too.

I decided not to say anything for now.

And see how they've replanted this garden area?

Oh, Mom, I'd forgotten how pretty the river is!

Isn't it just wonderful?

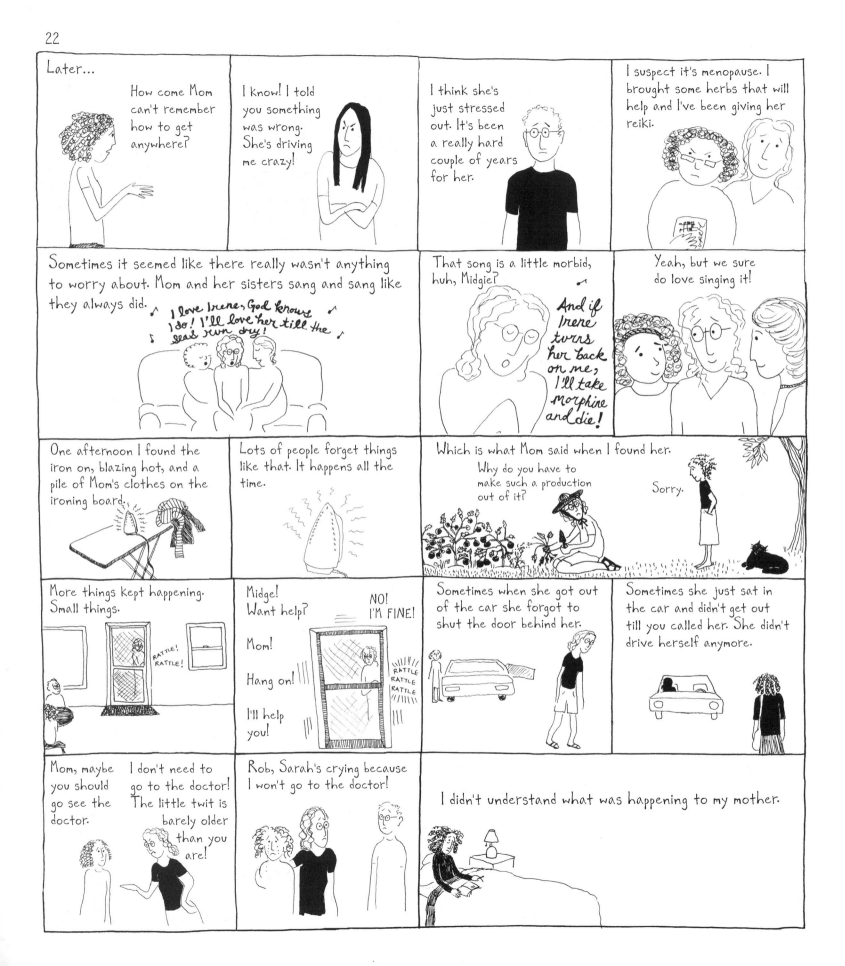

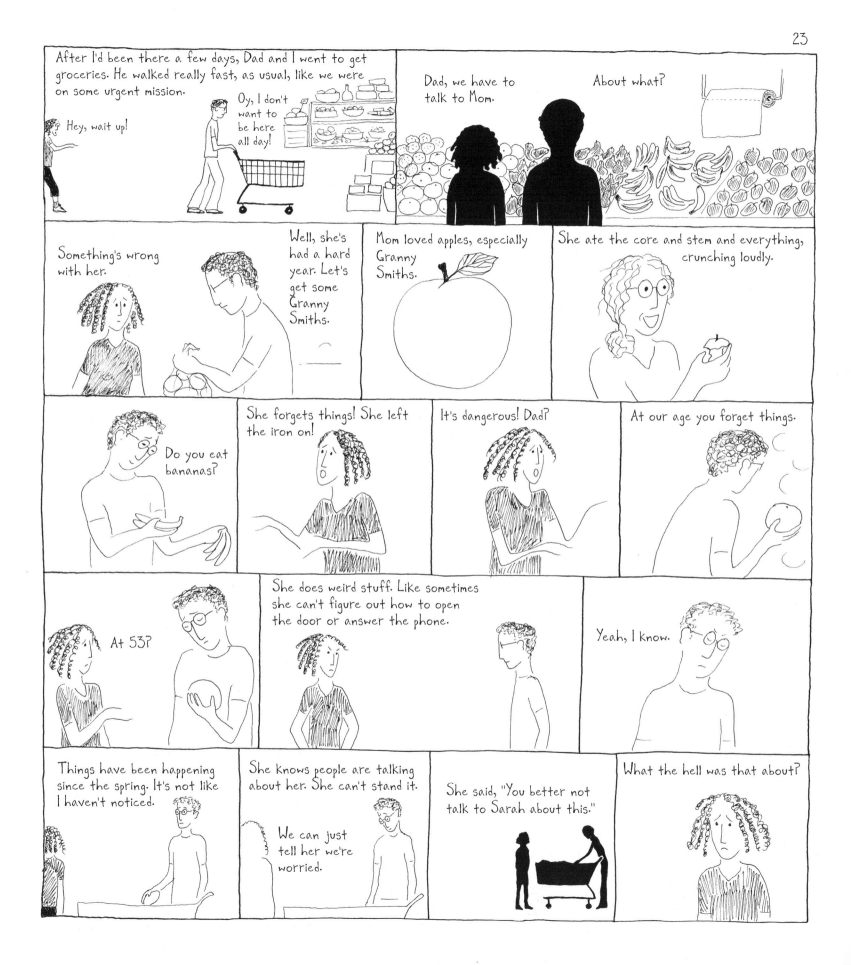

24

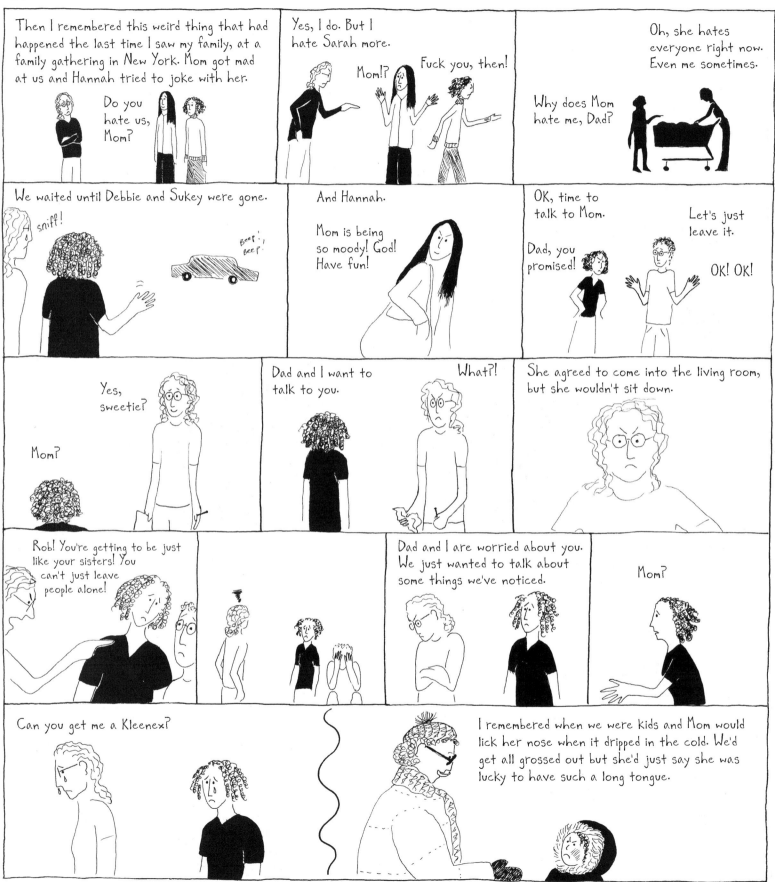

Panel 1: Then I remembered this weird thing that had happened the last time I saw my family, at a family gathering in New York. Mom got mad at us and Hannah tried to joke with her.
Do you hate us, Mom?

Panel 2: Yes, I do. But I hate Sarah more.
Mom!?
Fuck you, then!

Panel 3: Oh, she hates everyone right now. Even me sometimes.
Why does Mom hate me, Dad?

Panel 4: We waited until Debbie and Sukey were gone.
sniff!
Beep! Beep!

Panel 5: And Hannah.
Mom is being so moody! God! Have fun!

Panel 6: OK, time to talk to Mom.
Let's just leave it.
Dad, you promised!
OK! OK!

Panel 7: Mom?
Yes, sweetie?

Panel 8: Dad and I want to talk to you.
What?!

Panel 9: She agreed to come into the living room, but she wouldn't sit down.

Panel 10: Rob! You're getting to be just like your sisters! You can't just leave people alone!

Panel 11: (no text)

Panel 12: Dad and I are worried about you. We just wanted to talk about some things we've noticed.

Panel 13: Mom?

Panel 14: Can you get me a Kleenex?

Panel 15: I remembered when we were kids and Mom would lick her nose when it dripped in the cold. We'd get all grossed out but she'd just say she was lucky to have such a long tongue.

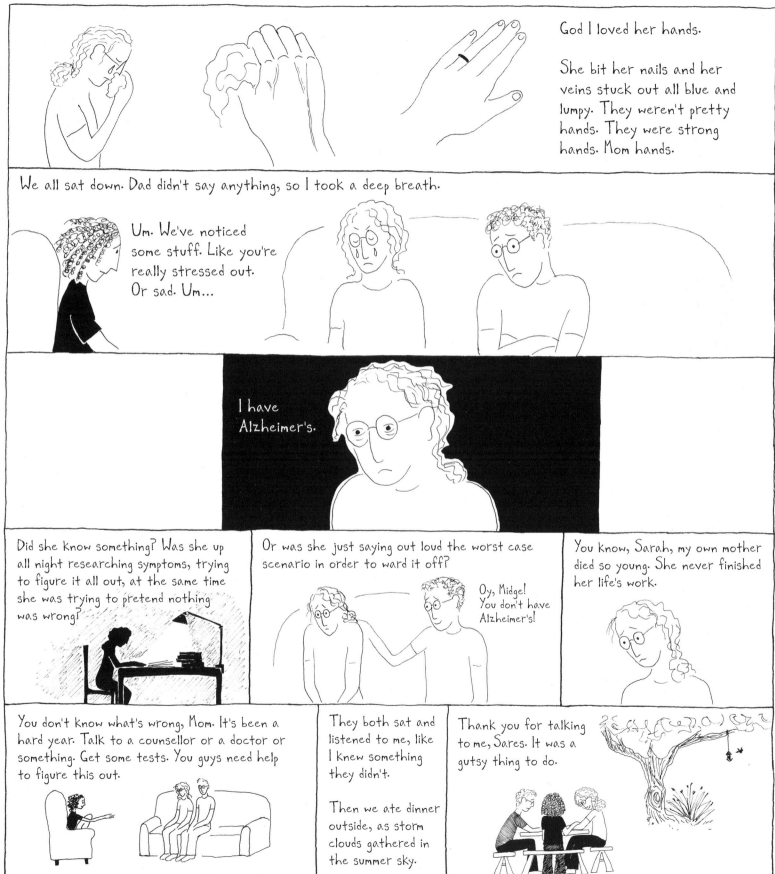

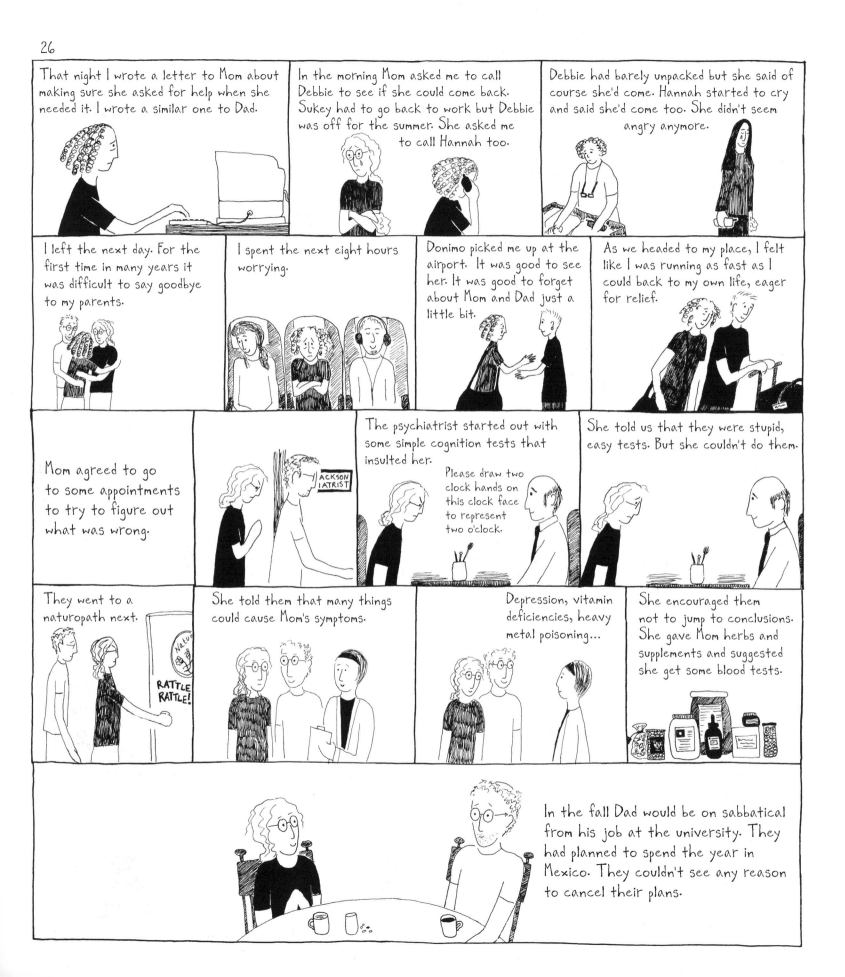

That night I wrote a letter to Mom about making sure she asked for help when she needed it. I wrote a similar one to Dad.

In the morning Mom asked me to call Debbie to see if she could come back. Sukey had to go back to work but Debbie was off for the summer. She asked me to call Hannah too.

Debbie had barely unpacked but she said of course she'd come. Hannah started to cry and said she'd come too. She didn't seem angry anymore.

I left the next day. For the first time in many years it was difficult to say goodbye to my parents.

I spent the next eight hours worrying.

Donimo picked me up at the airport. It was good to see her. It was good to forget about Mom and Dad just a little bit.

As we headed to my place, I felt like I was running as fast as I could back to my own life, eager for relief.

Mom agreed to go to some appointments to try to figure out what was wrong.

ACKSON IATRIST

The psychiatrist started out with some simple cognition tests that insulted her.

Please draw two clock hands on this clock face to represent two o'clock.

She told us that they were stupid, easy tests. But she couldn't do them.

They went to a naturopath next.

RATTLE RATTLE!

She told them that many things could cause Mom's symptoms.

Depression, vitamin deficiencies, heavy metal poisoning...

She encouraged them not to jump to conclusions. She gave Mom herbs and supplements and suggested she get some blood tests.

In the fall Dad would be on sabbatical from his job at the university. They had planned to spend the year in Mexico. They couldn't see any reason to cancel their plans.

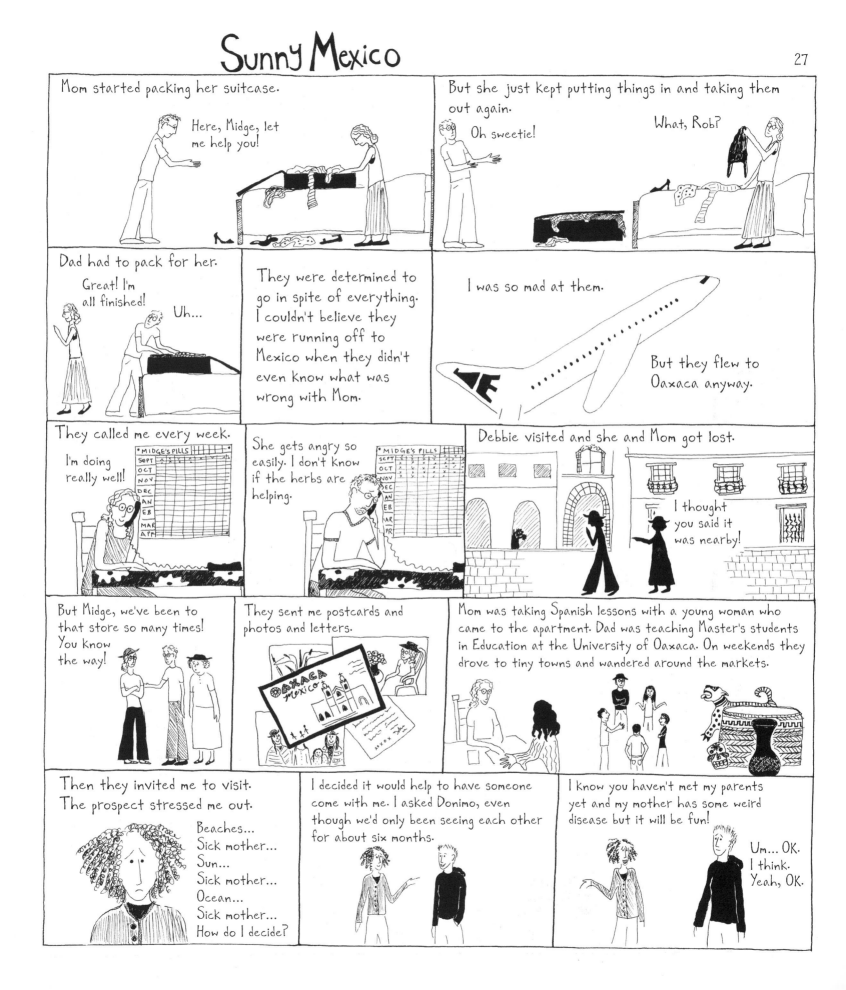

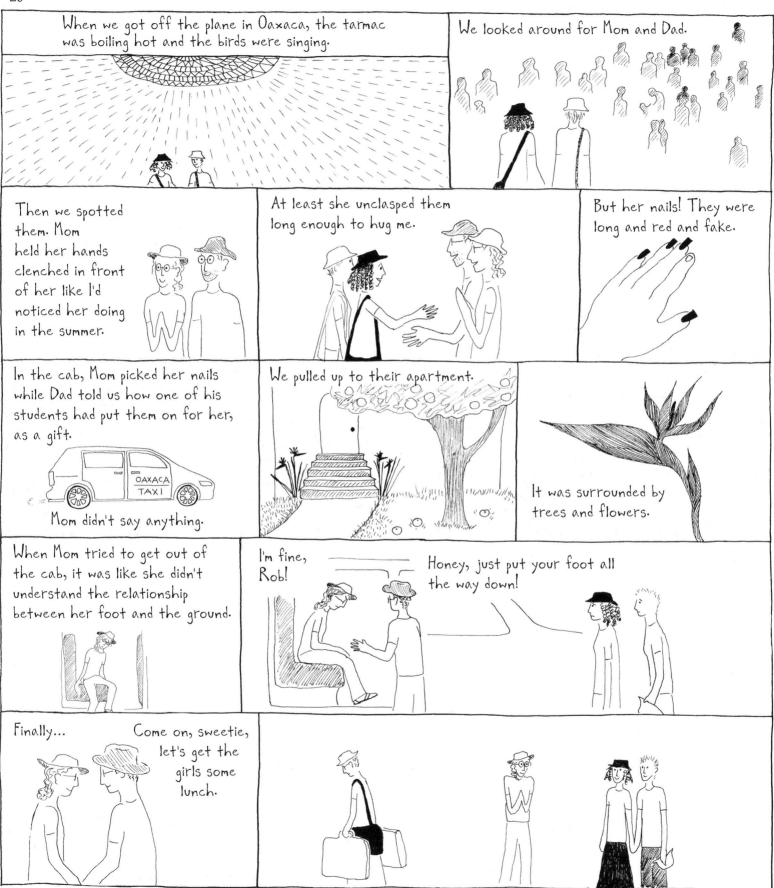

When we got off the plane in Oaxaca, the tarmac was boiling hot and the birds were singing.

We looked around for Mom and Dad.

Then we spotted them. Mom held her hands clenched in front of her like I'd noticed her doing in the summer.

At least she unclasped them long enough to hug me.

But her nails! They were long and red and fake.

In the cab, Mom picked her nails while Dad told us how one of his students had put them on for her, as a gift.

OAXACA TAXI

Mom didn't say anything.

We pulled up to their apartment.

It was surrounded by trees and flowers.

When Mom tried to get out of the cab, it was like she didn't understand the relationship between her foot and the ground.

I'm fine, Rob!

Honey, just put your foot all the way down!

Finally...

Come on, sweetie, let's get the girls some lunch.

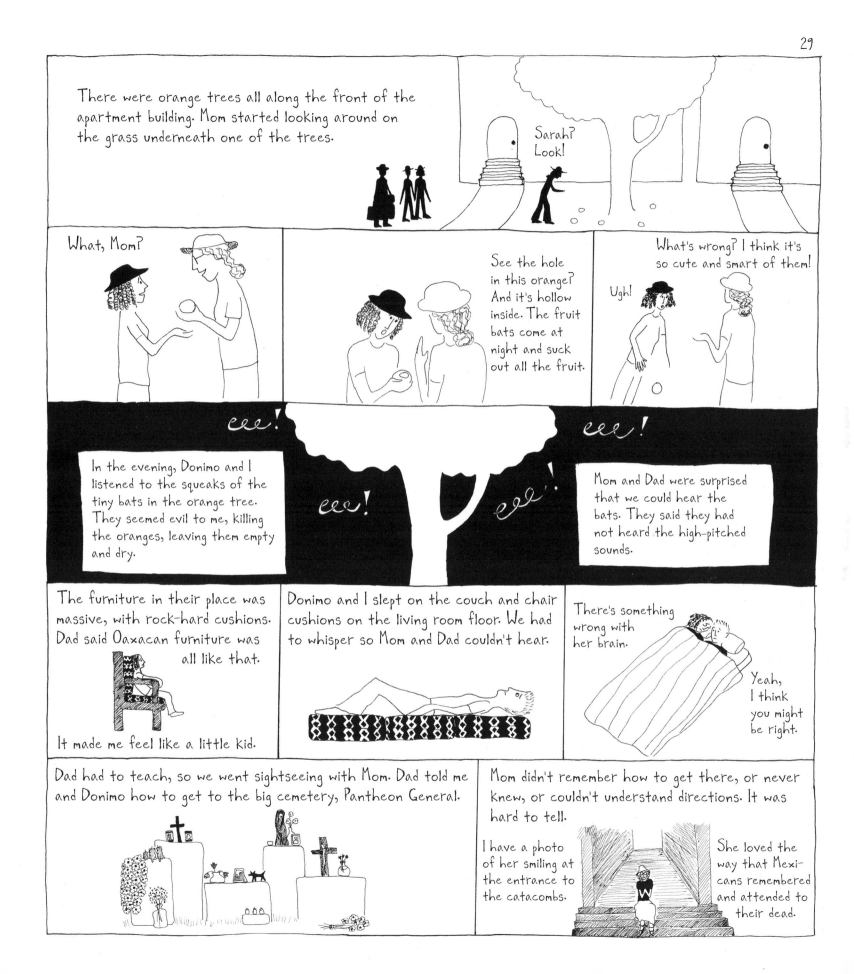

There were orange trees all along the front of the apartment building. Mom started looking around on the grass underneath one of the trees.

Sarah? Look!

What, Mom?

See the hole in this orange? And it's hollow inside. The fruit bats come at night and suck out all the fruit.

Ugh!

What's wrong? I think it's so cute and smart of them!

eee!   eee!   eee!   eee!

In the evening, Donimo and I listened to the squeaks of the tiny bats in the orange tree. They seemed evil to me, killing the oranges, leaving them empty and dry.

Mom and Dad were surprised that we could hear the bats. They said they had not heard the high-pitched sounds.

The furniture in their place was massive, with rock-hard cushions. Dad said Oaxacan furniture was all like that.

It made me feel like a little kid.

Donimo and I slept on the couch and chair cushions on the living room floor. We had to whisper so Mom and Dad couldn't hear.

There's something wrong with her brain.

Yeah, I think you might be right.

Dad had to teach, so we went sightseeing with Mom. Dad told me and Donimo how to get to the big cemetery, Pantheon General.

Mom didn't remember how to get there, or never knew, or couldn't understand directions. It was hard to tell.

I have a photo of her smiling at the entrance to the catacombs.

She loved the way that Mexicans remembered and attended to their dead.

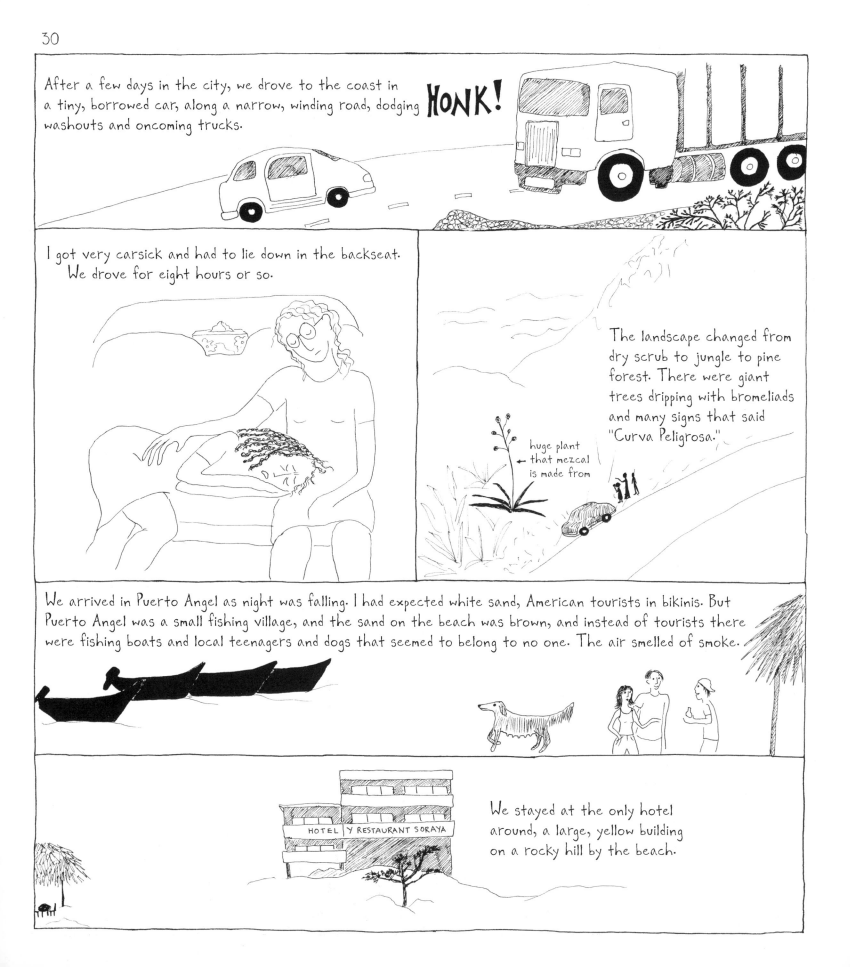

After a few days in the city, we drove to the coast in a tiny, borrowed car, along a narrow, winding road, dodging washouts and oncoming trucks.

HONK!

I got very carsick and had to lie down in the backseat. We drove for eight hours or so.

The landscape changed from dry scrub to jungle to pine forest. There were giant trees dripping with bromeliads and many signs that said "Curva Peligrosa."

huge plant ← that mezcal is made from

We arrived in Puerto Angel as night was falling. I had expected white sand, American tourists in bikinis. But Puerto Angel was a small fishing village, and the sand on the beach was brown, and instead of tourists there were fishing boats and local teenagers and dogs that seemed to belong to no one. The air smelled of smoke.

HOTEL Y RESTAURANT SORAYA

We stayed at the only hotel around, a large, yellow building on a rocky hill by the beach.

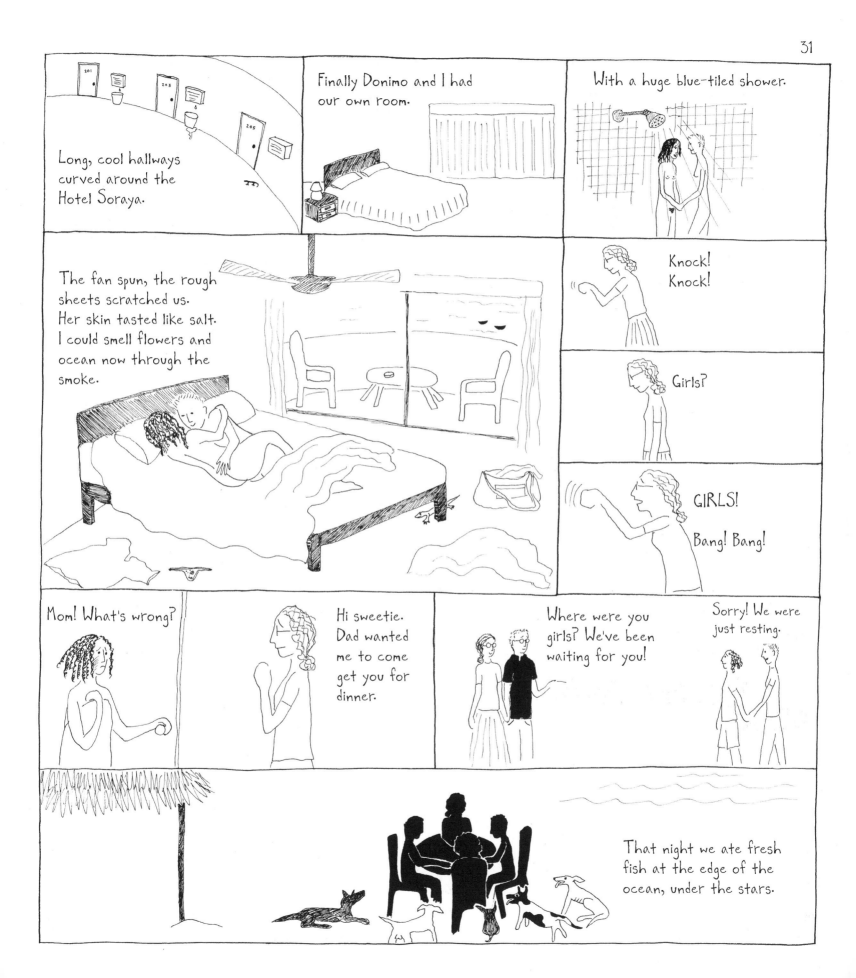

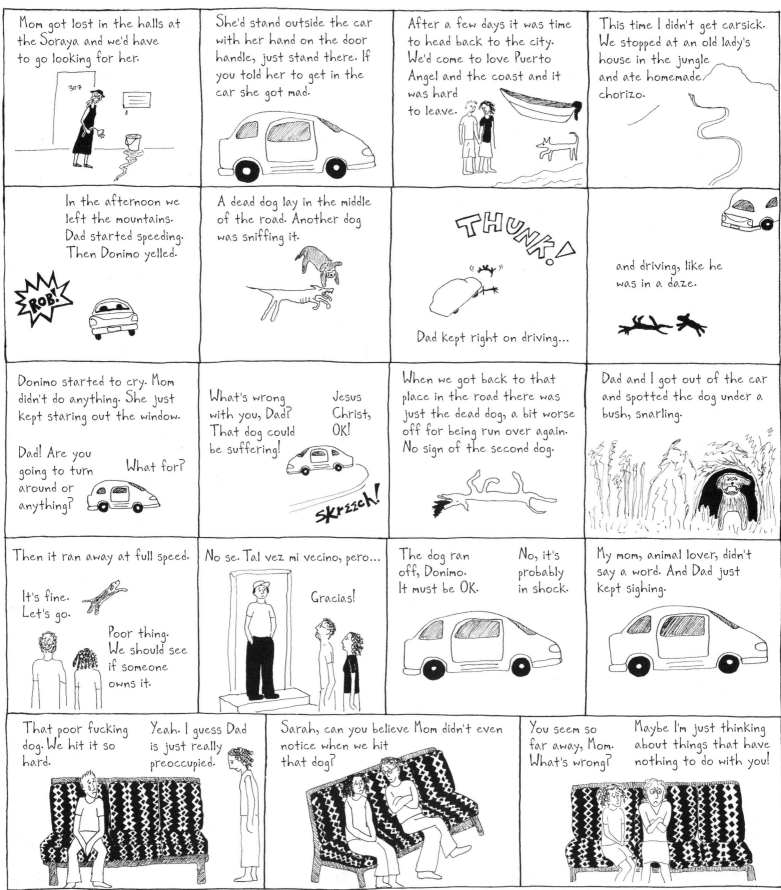

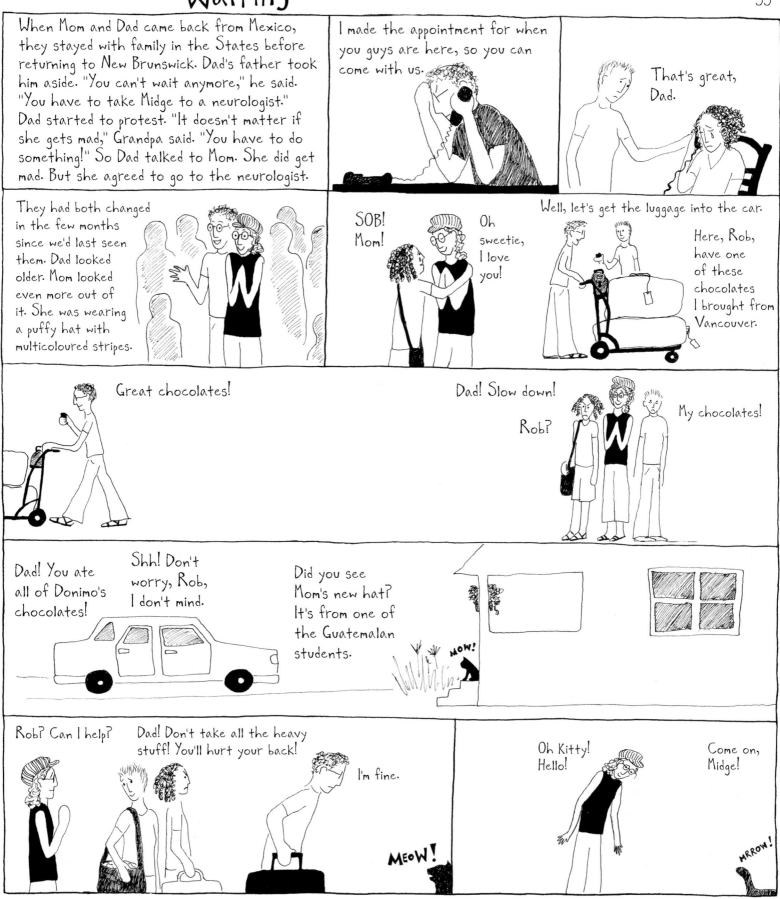

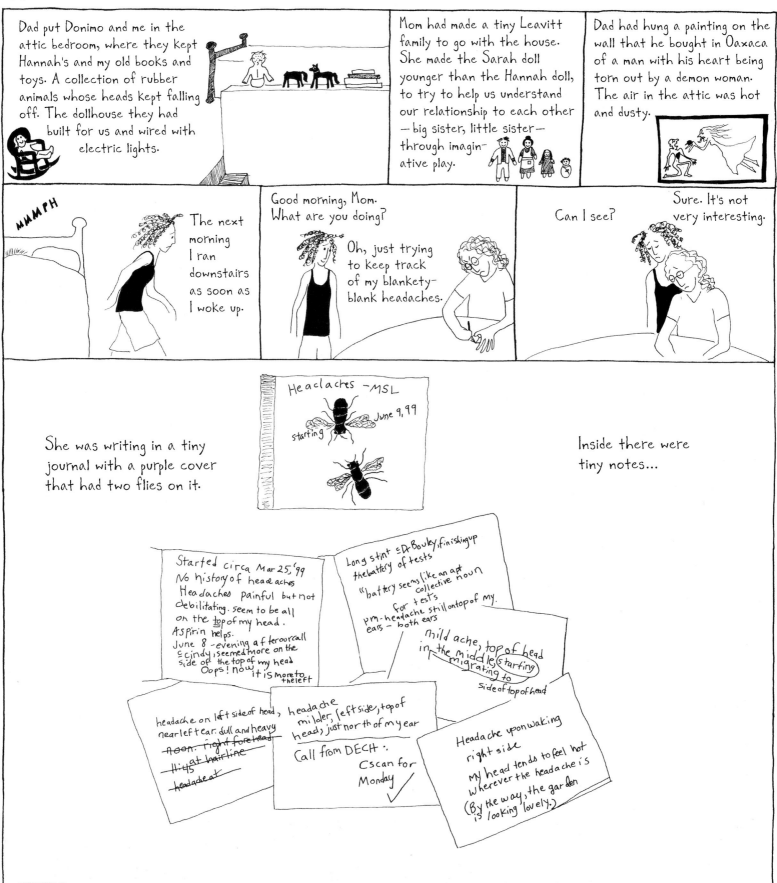

Dad put Donimo and me in the attic bedroom, where they kept Hannah's and my old books and toys. A collection of rubber animals whose heads kept falling off. The dollhouse they had built for us and wired with electric lights.

Mom had made a tiny Leavitt family to go with the house. She made the Sarah doll younger than the Hannah doll, to try to help us understand our relationship to each other — big sister, little sister — through imaginative play.

Dad had hung a painting on the wall that he bought in Oaxaca of a man with his heart being torn out by a demon woman. The air in the attic was hot and dusty.

MMMPH

The next morning I ran downstairs as soon as I woke up.

Good morning, Mom. What are you doing?

Oh, just trying to keep track of my blankety-blank headaches.

Can I see?

Sure. It's not very interesting.

Headaches —MSL
starting   June 9, 99

She was writing in a tiny journal with a purple cover that had two flies on it.

Inside there were tiny notes...

Started circa Mar 25, '99
No history of headaches
Headaches painful but not debilitating. seem to be all on the top of my head.
Aspirin helps.
June 8 - evening after our call with cindy, seemed more on the side of the top of my head
Oops! now it is more to the left

Long stint at Bouky, finishing up the battery of tests
"battery seems like an apt collective noun for tests
pm - headache still on top of my ears — both ears
mild ache, top of head in the middle, starting to migrating to side of top of head

headache on left side of head, near left ear. dull and heavy
Noon. right forehead
Hit at hairline
headache at

headache milder, left side, top of head, just north of my ear
Call from DECH:
C scan for Monday ✓

Headache upon waking right side
My head tends to feel hot wherever the headache is
(By the way, the garden is looking lovely.)

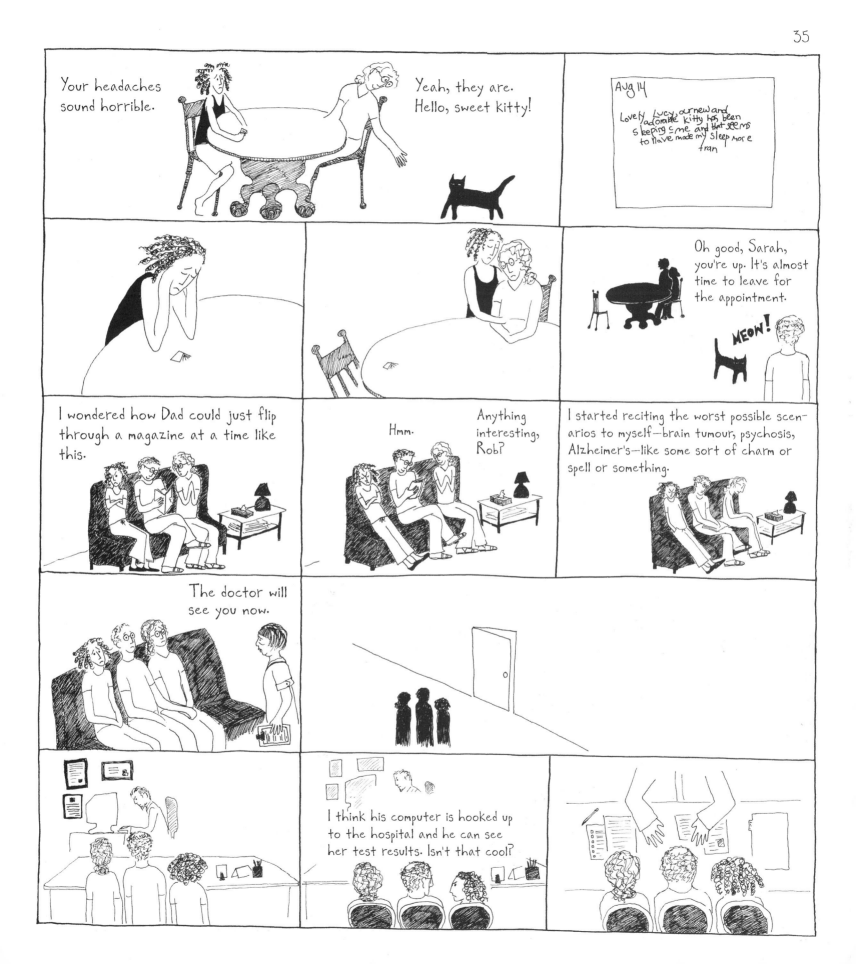

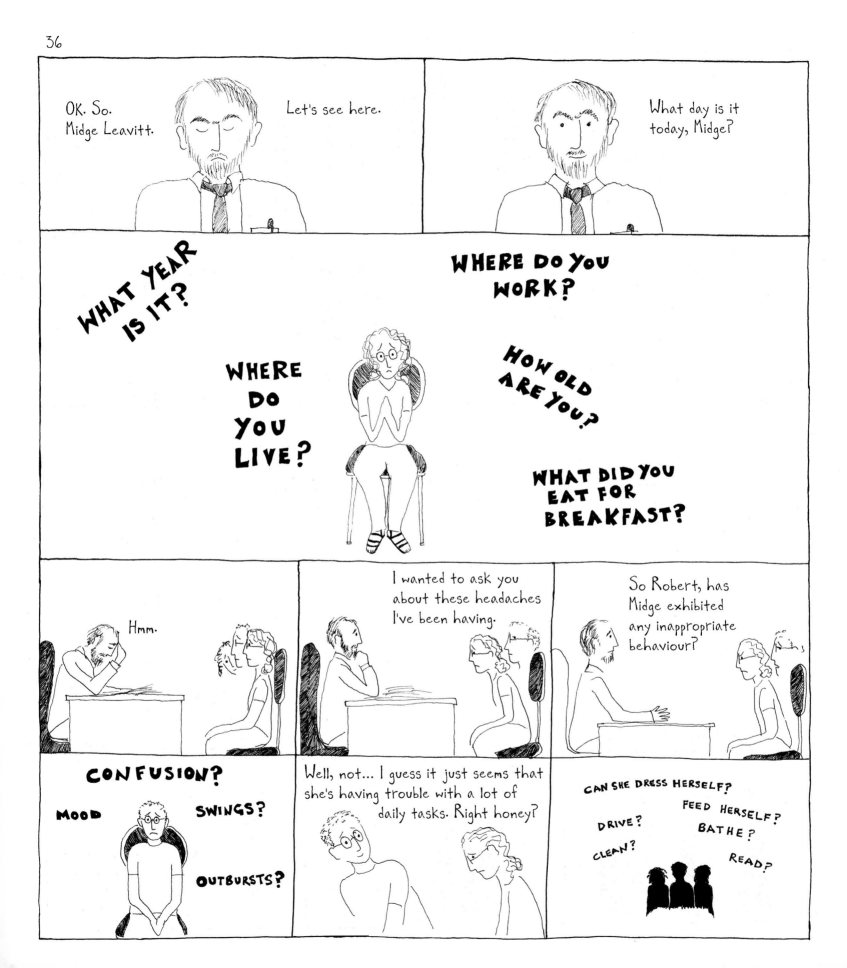

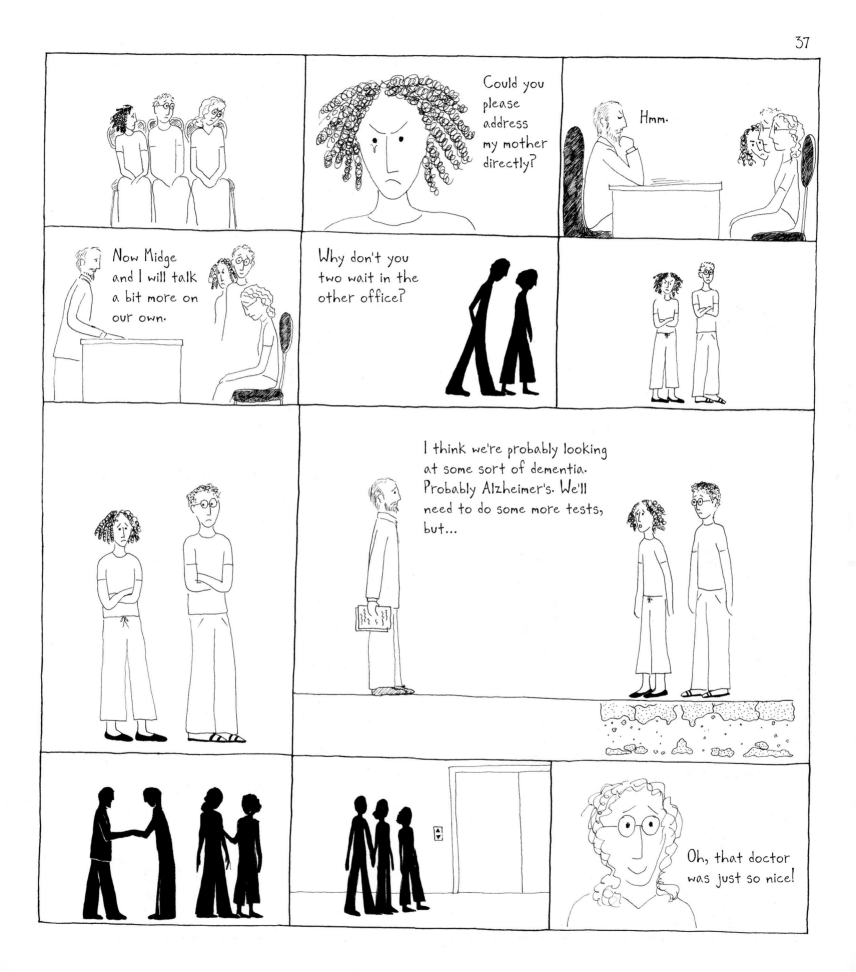

Language

Mom started at Radcliffe College in 1962. She was very cool.

She wore a genuine peacoat and she smoked.

She met Dad, a Harvard student, in their final year. They always laughed about how well-behaved and naive they both were.

They each got drunk once in college. Mom spent an evening on top of a refrigerator.

Dad walked across Harvard Yard barefoot in the winter.

A few months after they started dating, Dad gave Mom an engagement ring he'd made himself, a copper band that turned her finger green.

They had a small wedding. Dad's sisters cried to see him go, and Mom always held it against them.

They had two kids and moved to the country...

where they built a life of books and art and creativity. They never owned a television.

Hannah and I grew up surrounded by beloved characters from our favourite books, from Oz, Narnia, Middle Earth, Moominland.

TIK-TOK OF OZ

Many of them seemed like our intimate friends.

SNUFKIN

We all loved The Lord of the Rings. The Black Riders terrified us.

Dad and I cried together when Gandalf died.

We also read all the Little House on the Prairie books. Mom made us old-fashioned outfits so we could dress up like Laura and Mary Ingalls.

Mom and Dad must have read to us almost every day of our childhoods.

They also loved making up nicknames for us, especially Dad. I was Sarah Beanstalk for Sarah Beatrice, and Large Brown Woman for some unknown reason.

Hannah was Hanner, because that's how they said it in Maine, and 14 Women for no reason, and Wim because it was short for 14 Women.

Dad was RML, his initials, and Mom was many things, including Migdel, a variation of Midge, which then became Mrs. Migdelpopper.

Our first cat, Emily, was Beelzebub or Beels or Kitten Kaboodle.

In junior high, Hannah took our language play to the next level with a collection of acronyms and made-up words that were so apt that Dad and Mom and I adopted many of them for our own use. Like if a couple was having an overly affectionate goodbye, we'd say they were being "piss," short for "parting is such sweet sorrow."

Dear Sarah,
I hope you are ha
She is HTP so
and then it was
bozzed up so
I said DP becau
all OTT and her
always P.I.S.S.

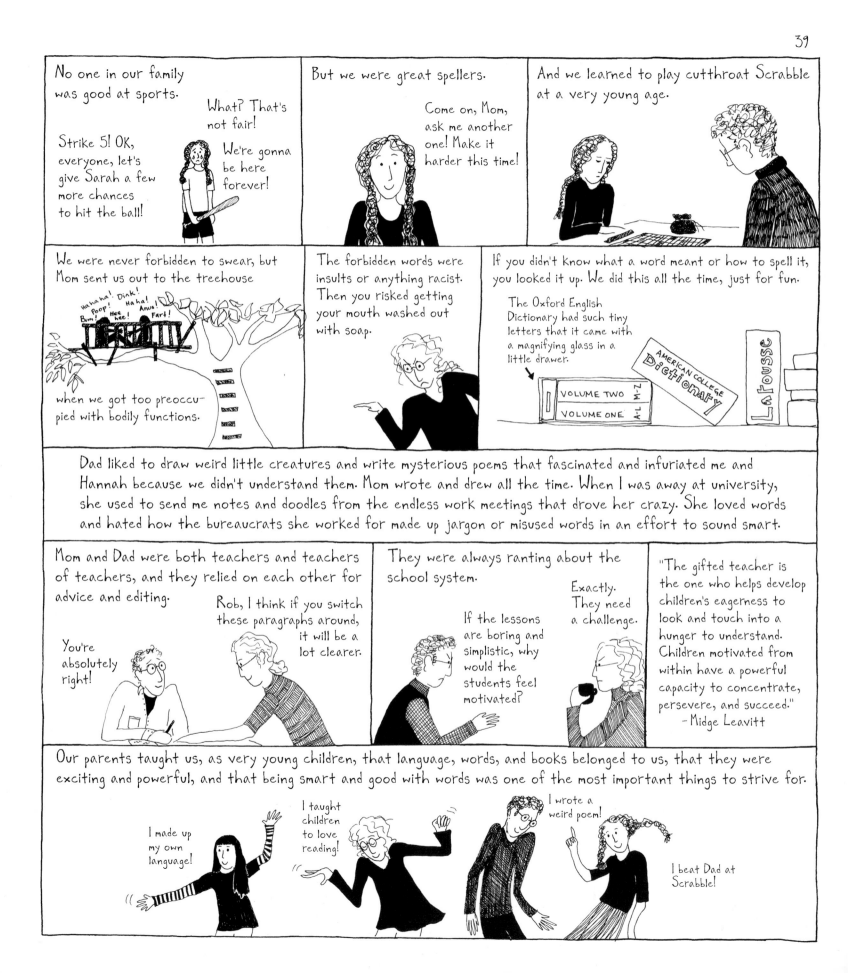

Diagnosis

That fall while we waited for the test results, Mom wrote to me a few times on index cards in marker. One letter included curling red maple leaves wrapped in a napkin.

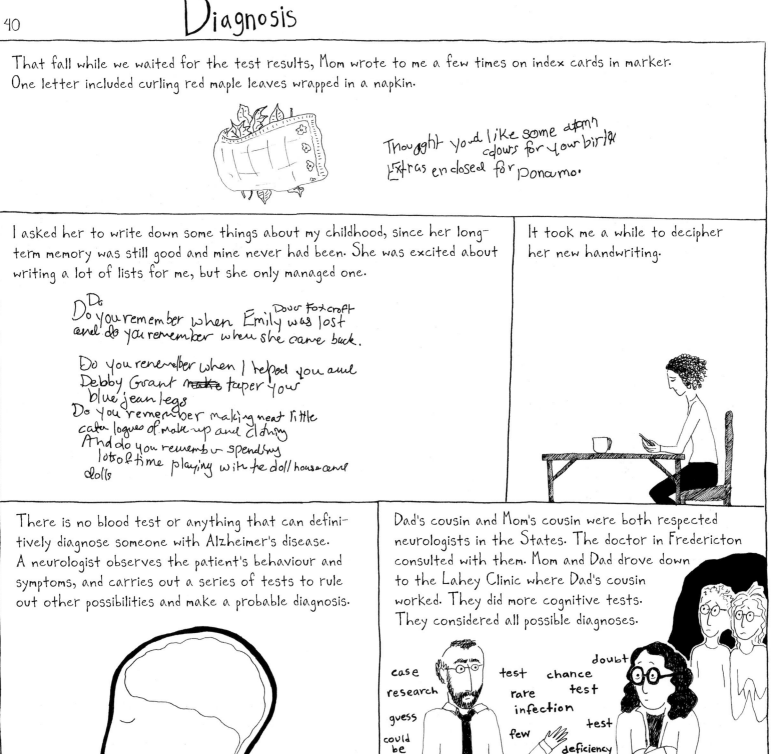

Thought you'd like some autumn colours for your birthday. Extras enclosed for Ponamo.

I asked her to write down some things about my childhood, since her long-term memory was still good and mine never had been. She was excited about writing a lot of lists for me, but she only managed one.

Do Do you remember when Emily Dover Foxcroft was lost and do you remember when she came back.

Do you remember when I helped you and Debby Grant make taper your blue jean legs
Do you remember making neat little catalogues of make-up and clothing
And do you remember spending lots of time playing with the doll house and dolls

It took me a while to decipher her new handwriting.

There is no blood test or anything that can definitively diagnose someone with Alzheimer's disease. A neurologist observes the patient's behaviour and symptoms, and carries out a series of tests to rule out other possibilities and make a probable diagnosis.

The only way to prove it was Alzheimer's was to do a brain biopsy, which was very painful, or to wait until an autopsy could be performed.

Dad's cousin and Mom's cousin were both respected neurologists in the States. The doctor in Fredericton consulted with them. Mom and Dad drove down to the Lahey Clinic where Dad's cousin worked. They did more cognitive tests. They considered all possible diagnoses.

case
research
guess
could
be
test
rare
infection
few
biopsy
maybe
chance
test
test
deficiency
test
small possibility
eliminate
percentage
indications
doubt
hope

Mom had an MRI, a CAT scan, and a PET scan. She didn't have a brain tumour or a blood clot or any signs of stroke.

She had a spinal tap, which ruled out some rare diseases of the central nervous system caused by tuberculosis and syphilis.

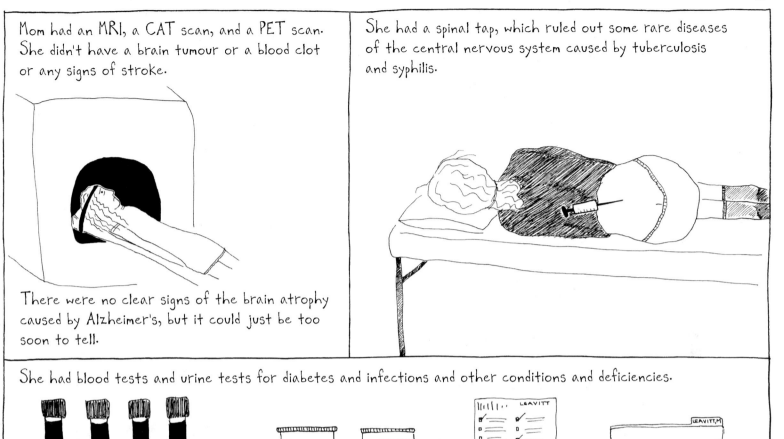

There were no clear signs of the brain atrophy caused by Alzheimer's, but it could just be too soon to tell.

She had blood tests and urine tests for diabetes and infections and other conditions and deficiencies.

The tests all came back negative. Dad's cousin said there was a chance that Mom could have a rare neurological disease that caused similar symptoms. But it was a miniscule chance and you could only tell for sure with a brain biopsy and the treatment was extremely painful and not guaranteed to work. Mom decided not to have the biopsy.

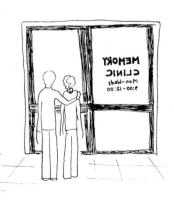

On October 6, 1999, Mom and Dad met with their neurologist. He said that all other possibilities had now been ruled out and the test results pointed to Alzheimer's. There was nothing else to try. Dad told me that as they left the clinic, he said to Mom, "It's not how we planned things, is it, Midge?"

He can't remember whether or not she answered him.

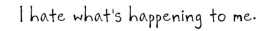

I hate what's happening to me.

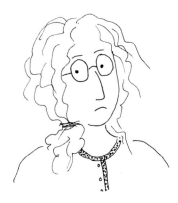

Part Two

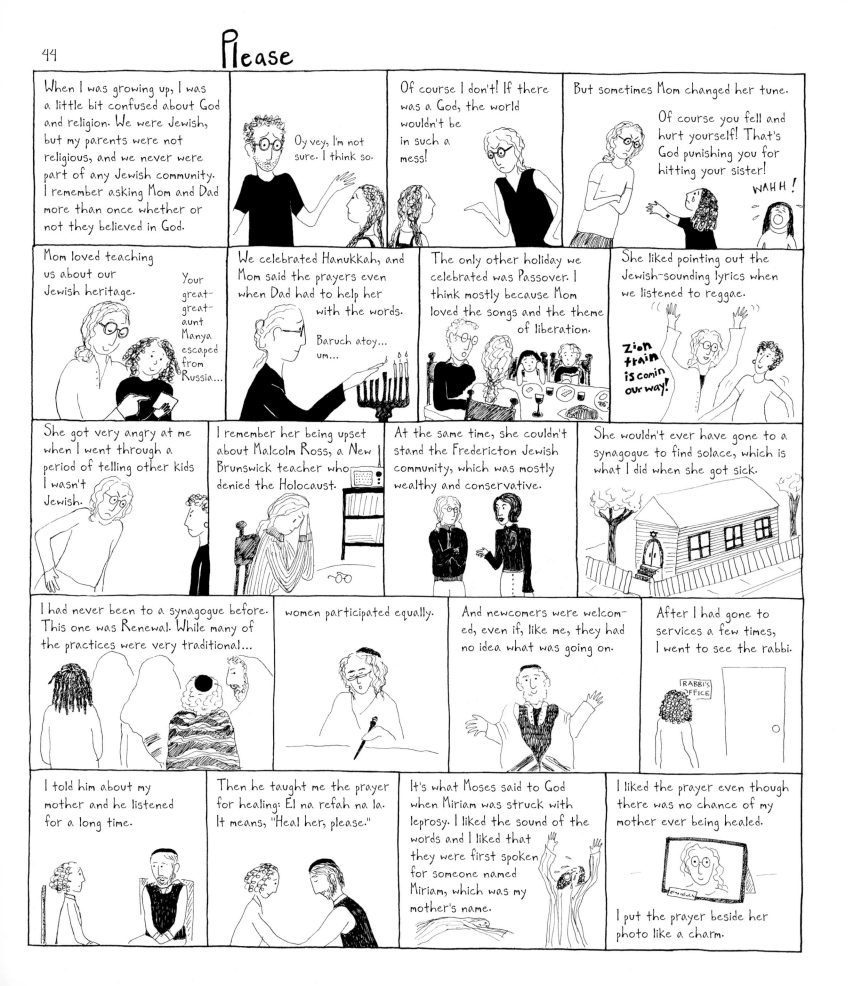

Please

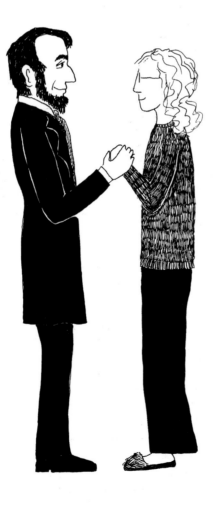

The Most Important

One time Mom was trying to tell us something.

She got very upset because she couldn't remember the name of the person she was talking about.

She kept repeating, "He was the most important!"

Dad kept trying to guess who it was, and finally he asked her if she was talking about Abraham Lincoln. "Yes!" she said, and started to cry.

Then she said to Dad, "That's right, right?"

"That people shouldn't have slaves?"

"Yes."

"Yes, sweetie. Of course that's right."

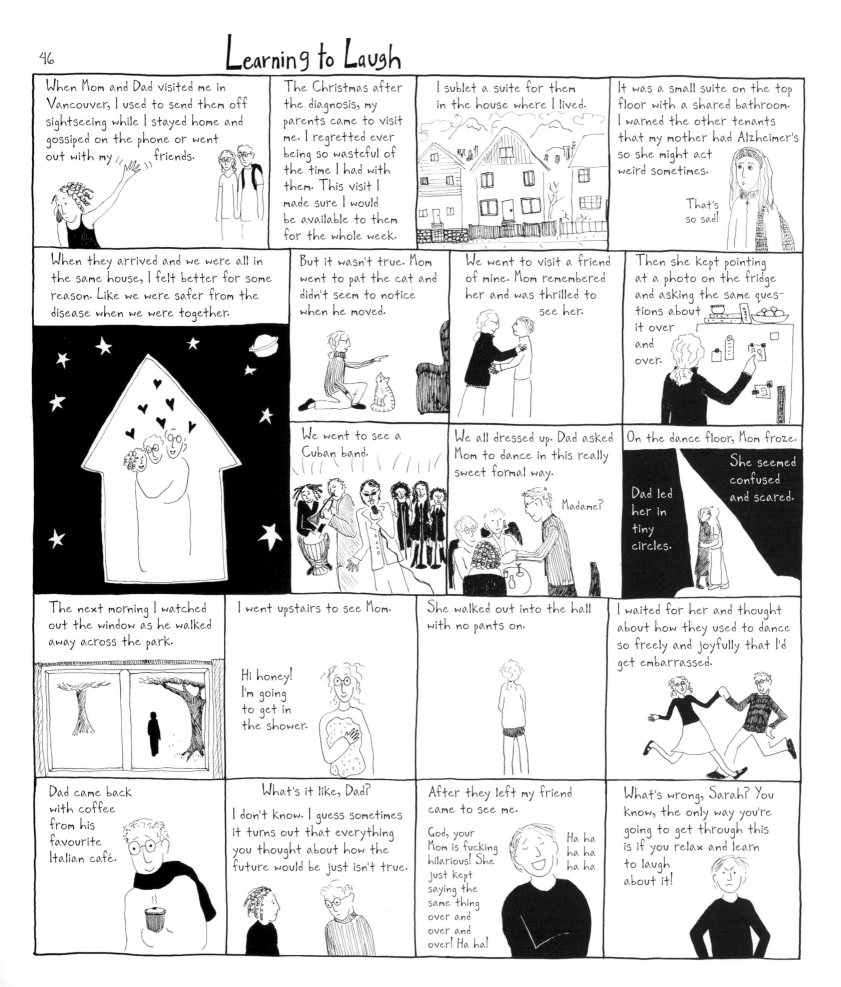

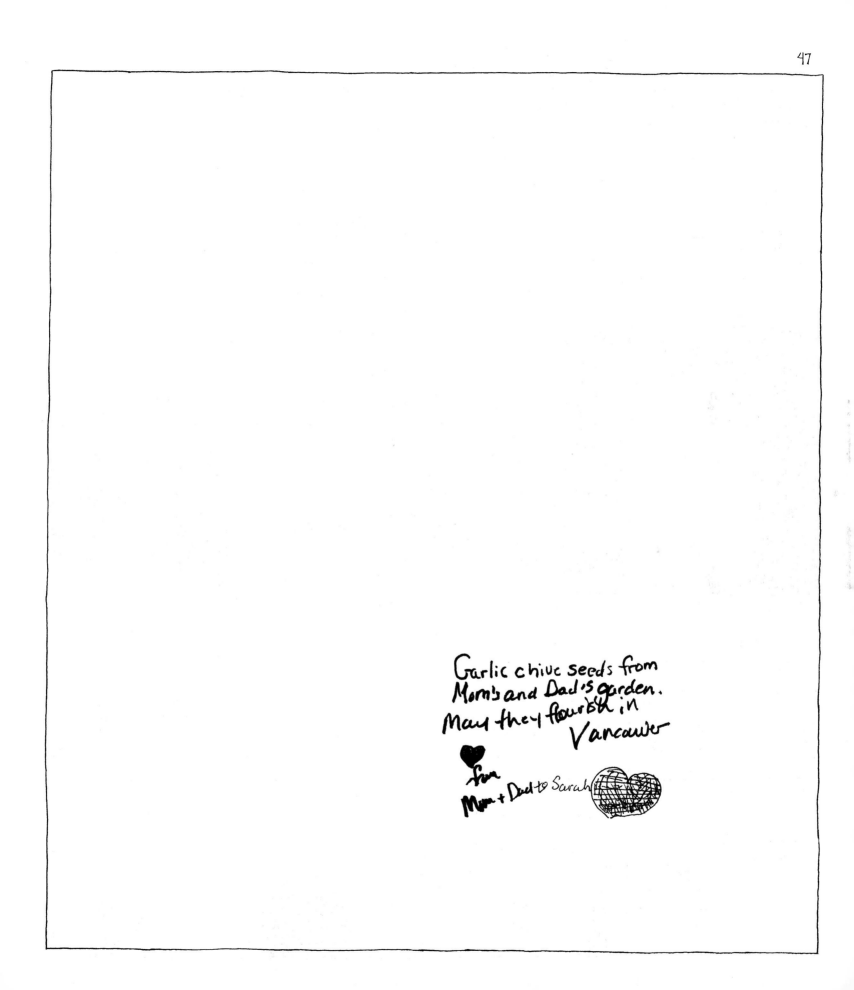

Garlic chive seeds from
Mom's and Dad's garden.
May they flourish in
Vancouver

from
Mom + Dad to Sarah

Shadowing

The next summer, Dad went back to Oaxaca for six weeks to visit and teach. He needed a break from Mom.

He had arranged with me and Debbie to stay with Mom while he was gone. We tried to act like we were coming to visit her, not to take care of her.

Debbie said she'd go for the first month.

I said I'd go for the last two weeks.

Hannah said she would visit, but she would not stay alone with Mom.

I'm just not like you and Debbie, OK? I'm not strong like you guys.

When I arrived some friends gave me a ride from the airport. It was almost midnight but the air was still thick and hot. I felt sick wondering what Mom would be like.

Midgie! Sarah's here! This way!

Hannah and Debbie gave me gifts for my 31st birthday, which had just passed. There was nothing from Mom and Dad. I tried not to pout. Mom and Dad had always showered us with gifts.

Mom had made me a card.

PS please help us to find a case for you and your flowers when they bloom

Debbie was doing her usual big sister bossy thing with Mom. I could see that Hannah was sick of it already. Mom didn't seem too happy either.

Debbie started updating me about distant relatives I had never met.

Hannah filled me in on her boyfriend and which girls were after him.

Mom just sat there.

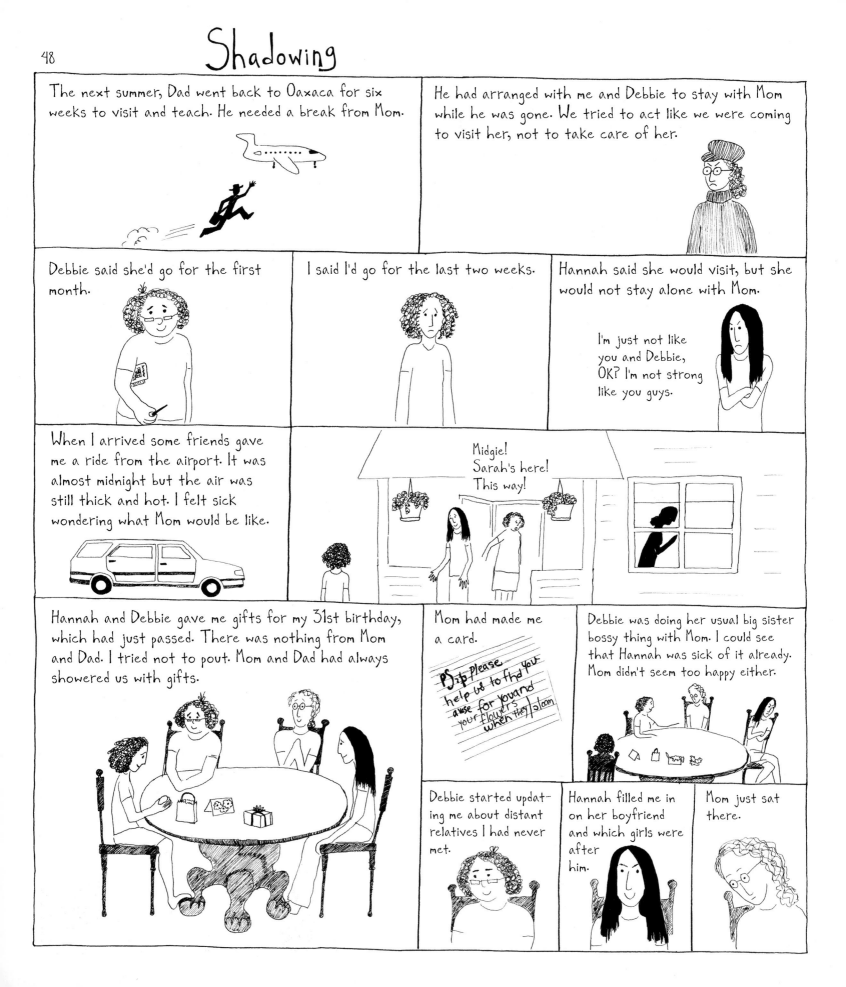

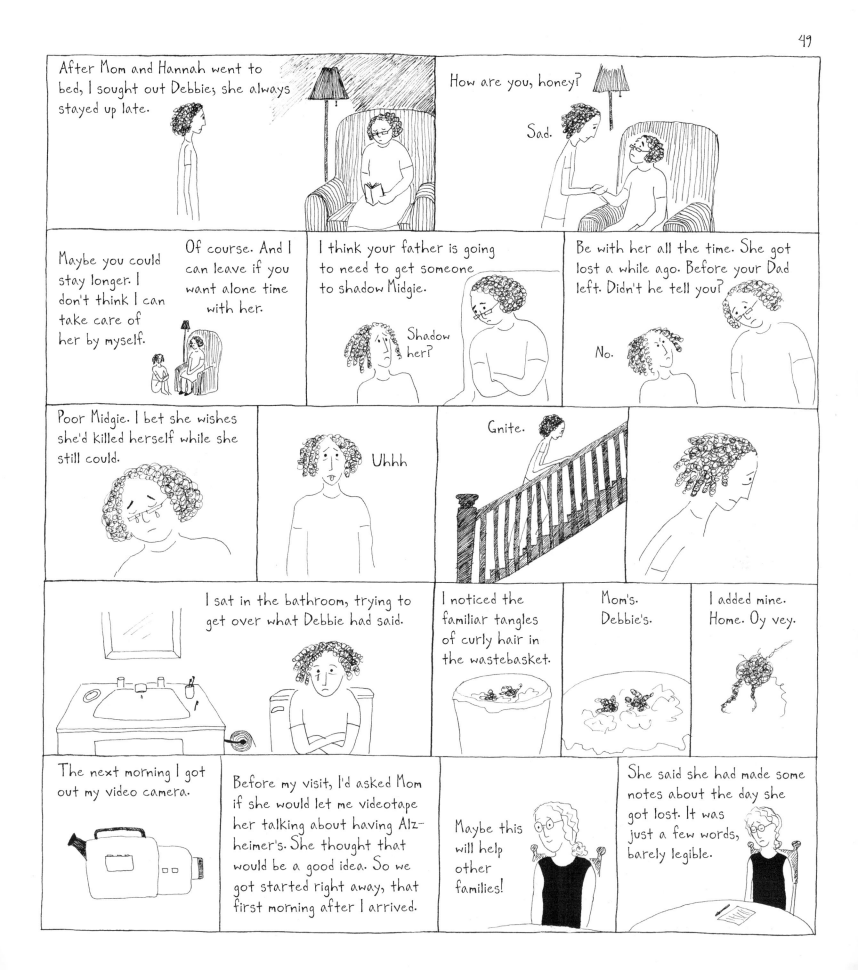

50

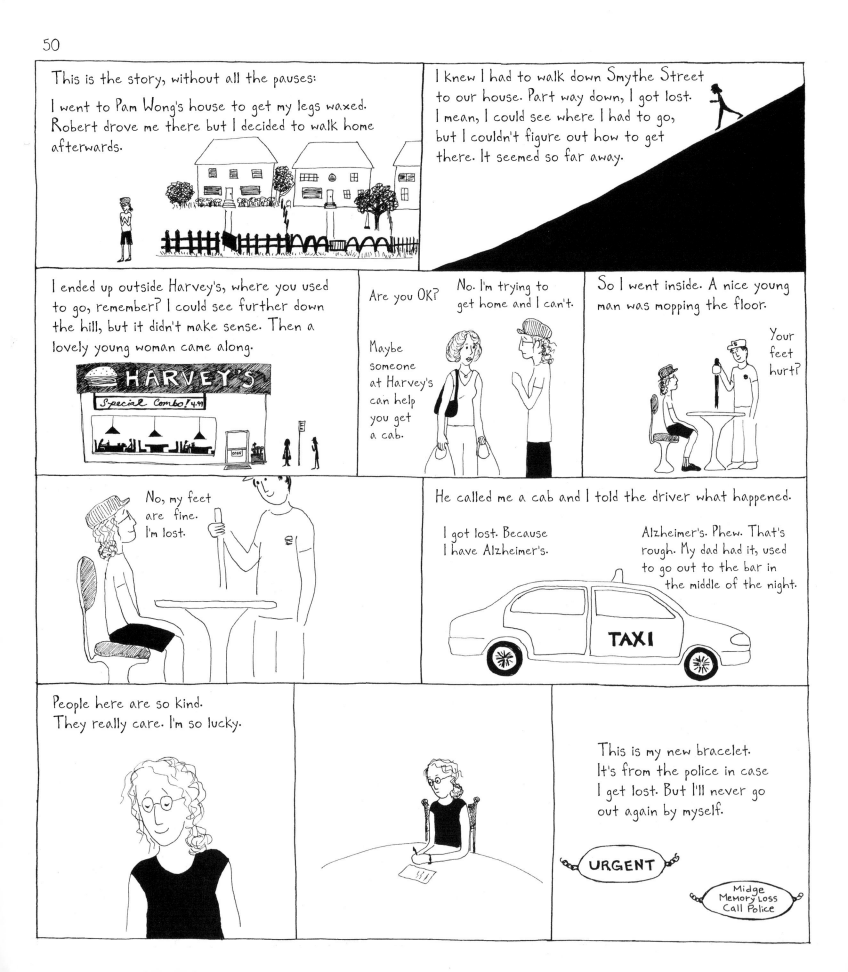

Food

When Hannah and I were growing up, Mom did her best to feed us healthy food. Like soup made from vegetables she'd grown from seed, and homemade bread.

Yuck!

I hate this!

After we moved out and had to fend for ourselves, we appreciated it more.

Welcome home, sweetie! I made some salad from the garden and muffins and...

Let's eat!

When Mom got sick, everything changed.

First the garden. Dad took on the planning and the soil preparation. He bought the seeds. Mom helped with weeding and harvesting.

But she couldn't manage to squat or kneel.

Even when she only meant to pull weeds, she pulled up lots of other plants too.

And she couldn't cook.

Tools became weapons.

Things got ruined.

Sometimes we'd give her a carrot and a dull knife and let her "help."

I miss... ten-pound loaves of dark rye, dense stews of vegetables grown from seed, with tofu mixed in to make it "proteinacious," a.k.a. "good 'n' good for you," honey carob cookies, homemade yoghurt...

rumble! growl!

Imagine, in the grief and silence of that house, Dad trying to cook for Mom.

Can I help, Rob?

No, it's OK.

Not that he couldn't cook. Far from it. Dad loved cooking as much as Mom did, though he was more likely to make treats.

← popovers for Sunday brunch

But when Mom got sick, he started making a lot of pasta with sauce from a jar.

Oh lovely! Thank you!

SPLAT!

Or they just didn't eat. Mom often didn't feel hunger (one of the effects of Alzheimer's), and Dad was probably just too depressed.

As Mom got sicker and their meals got smaller, I turned into some sort of...

extreme Jewish mother, obsessed with making them eat.

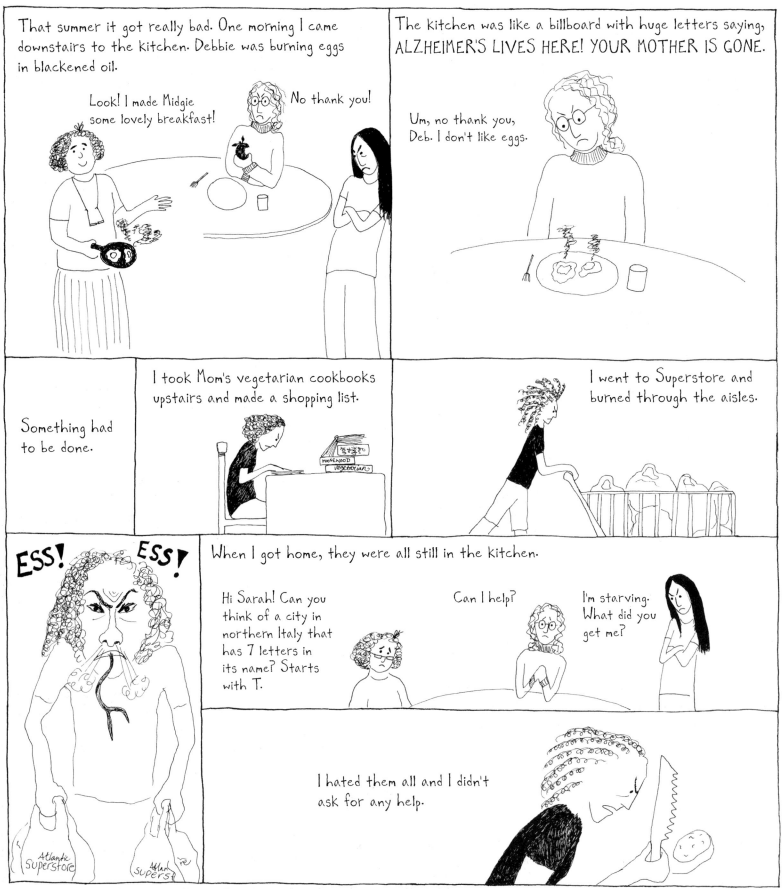

That summer it got really bad. One morning I came downstairs to the kitchen. Debbie was burning eggs in blackened oil.

Look! I made Midgie some lovely breakfast!

No thank you!

The kitchen was like a billboard with huge letters saying, ALZHEIMER'S LIVES HERE! YOUR MOTHER IS GONE.

Um, no thank you, Deb. I don't like eggs.

Something had to be done.

I took Mom's vegetarian cookbooks upstairs and made a shopping list.

MOOSEWOOD
vegetarian

I went to Superstore and burned through the aisles.

ESS! ESS!

Atlantic Superstore

When I got home, they were all still in the kitchen.

Hi Sarah! Can you think of a city in northern Italy that has 7 letters in its name? Starts with T.

Can I help?

I'm starving. What did you get me?

I hated them all and I didn't ask for any help.

Making the video was a great idea.

B U T

Mom would just sit there and not say anything.

Or she'd start crying.

She'd repeat over and over again this thing her dad said when he was dying of cancer: "I don't want there to be any secrets about my illness."

Ask me any questions you want! That's what Dad said and that's how it should be.

But the more questions I asked about how it was to have Alzheimer's, the quieter and angrier she got.

So I recorded her and Debbie reminiscing instead.

Deb, remember the stray cat that Mommy rescued?

One afternoon I played back some of the tape.

Mom watched in silence, looking more and more pissed off.

I guess my questions were kinda dumb, huh Mom?

No, it's that nicey-nice counsellor talk that you do!

We watched a bit more. Then...

That was great, Sarah! You really know how to let me be the expert. That's a rare skill.

Click!

Time to go up to the attic and eat gummy bears.

And cook huge meals.

And clean with a vengeance.

Mom wanted to help, but she couldn't, so she didn't.

Debbie sat on the couch and did puzzle after puzzle.

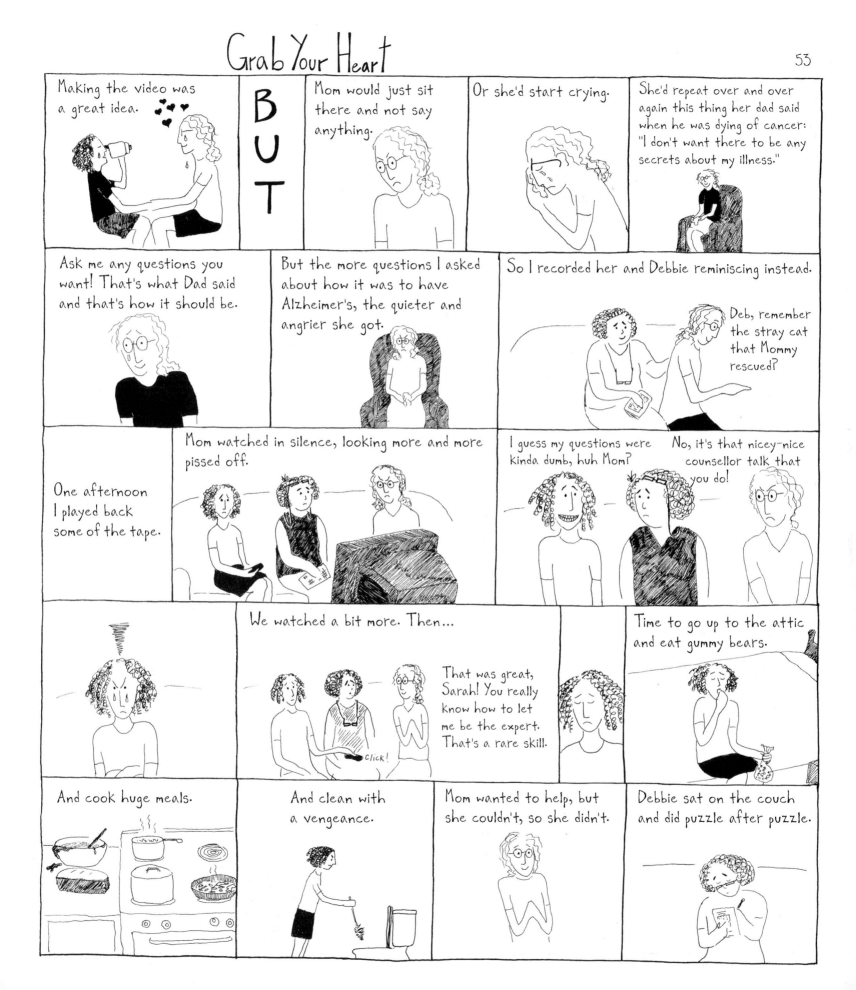

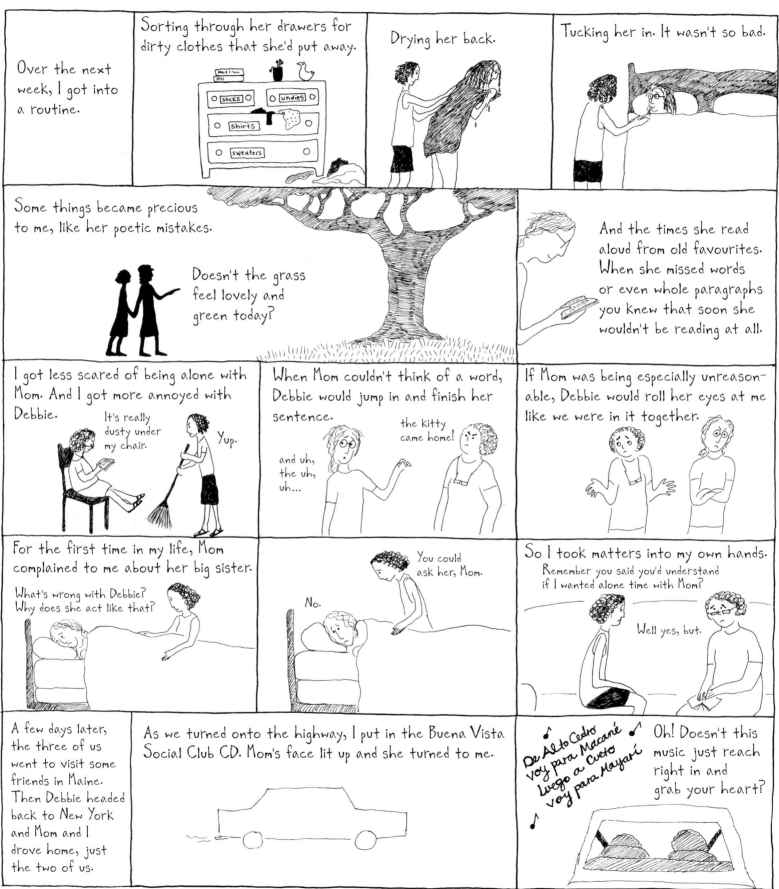

Over the next week, I got into a routine.

Sorting through her drawers for dirty clothes that she'd put away.

socks | undies
shirts
sweaters

Drying her back.

Tucking her in. It wasn't so bad.

Some things became precious to me, like her poetic mistakes.

Doesn't the grass feel lovely and green today?

And the times she read aloud from old favourites. When she missed words or even whole paragraphs you knew that soon she wouldn't be reading at all.

I got less scared of being alone with Mom. And I got more annoyed with Debbie.

It's really dusty under my chair.

Yup.

When Mom couldn't think of a word, Debbie would jump in and finish her sentence.

and uh, the uh, uh...

the kitty came home!

If Mom was being especially unreasonable, Debbie would roll her eyes at me like we were in it together.

For the first time in my life, Mom complained to me about her big sister.

What's wrong with Debbie? Why does she act like that?

You could ask her, Mom.

No.

So I took matters into my own hands.

Remember you said you'd understand if I wanted alone time with Mom?

Well yes, but.

A few days later, the three of us went to visit some friends in Maine. Then Debbie headed back to New York and Mom and I drove home, just the two of us.

As we turned onto the highway, I put in the Buena Vista Social Club CD. Mom's face lit up and she turned to me.

De Alto Cedro voy para Macané Luego a Cueto voy para Mayarí

Oh! Doesn't this music just reach right in and grab your heart?

Psycho Killer

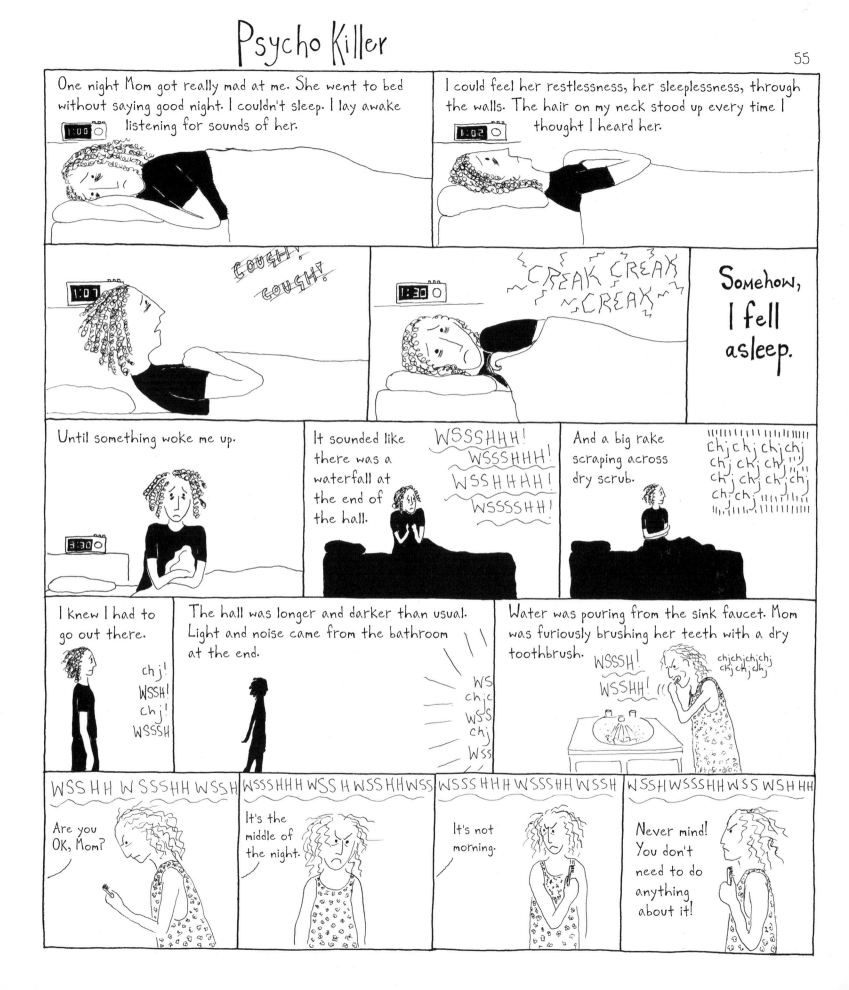

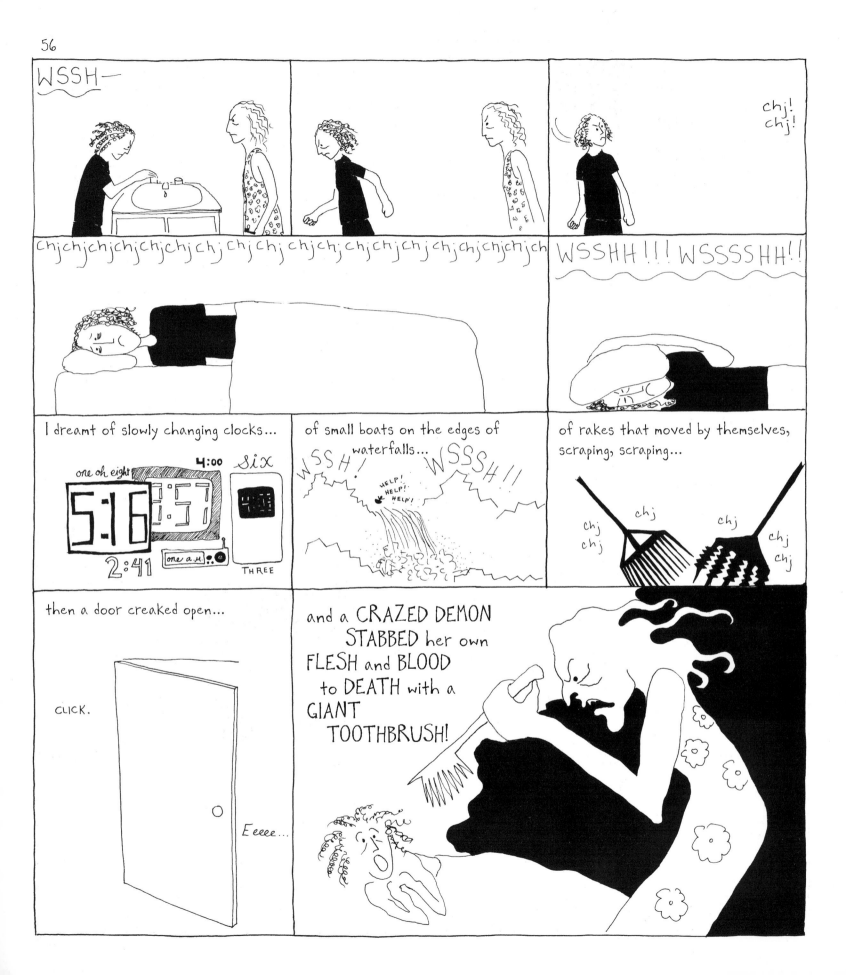

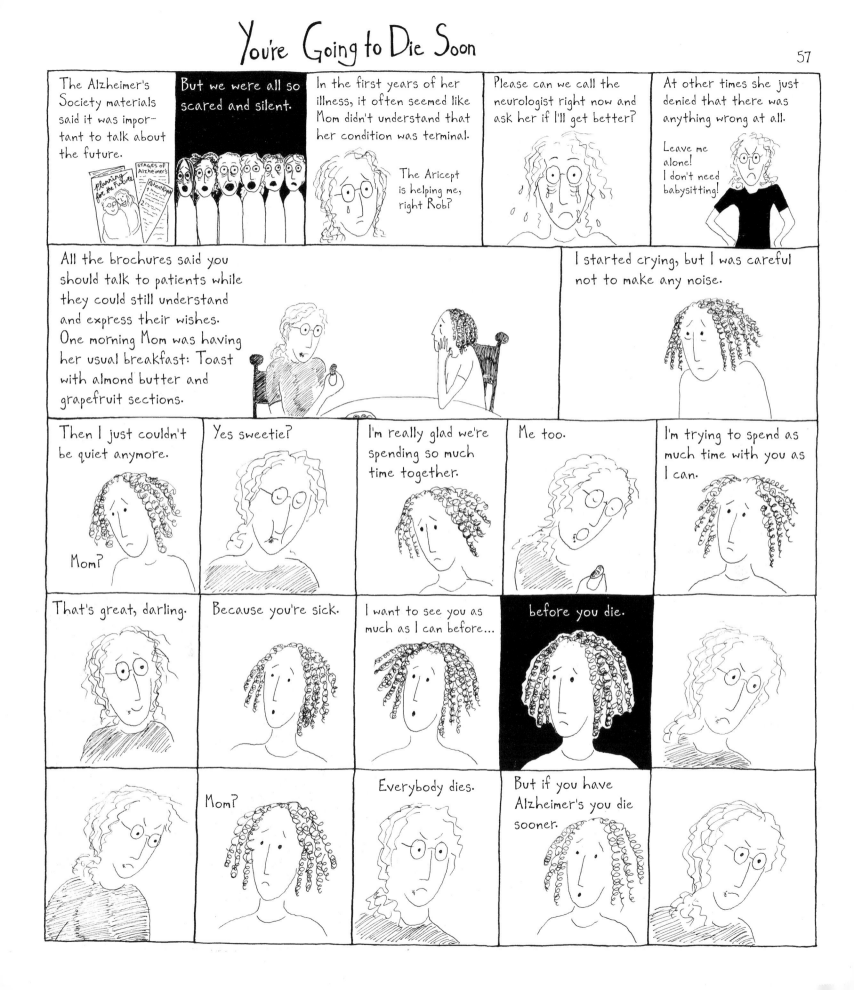

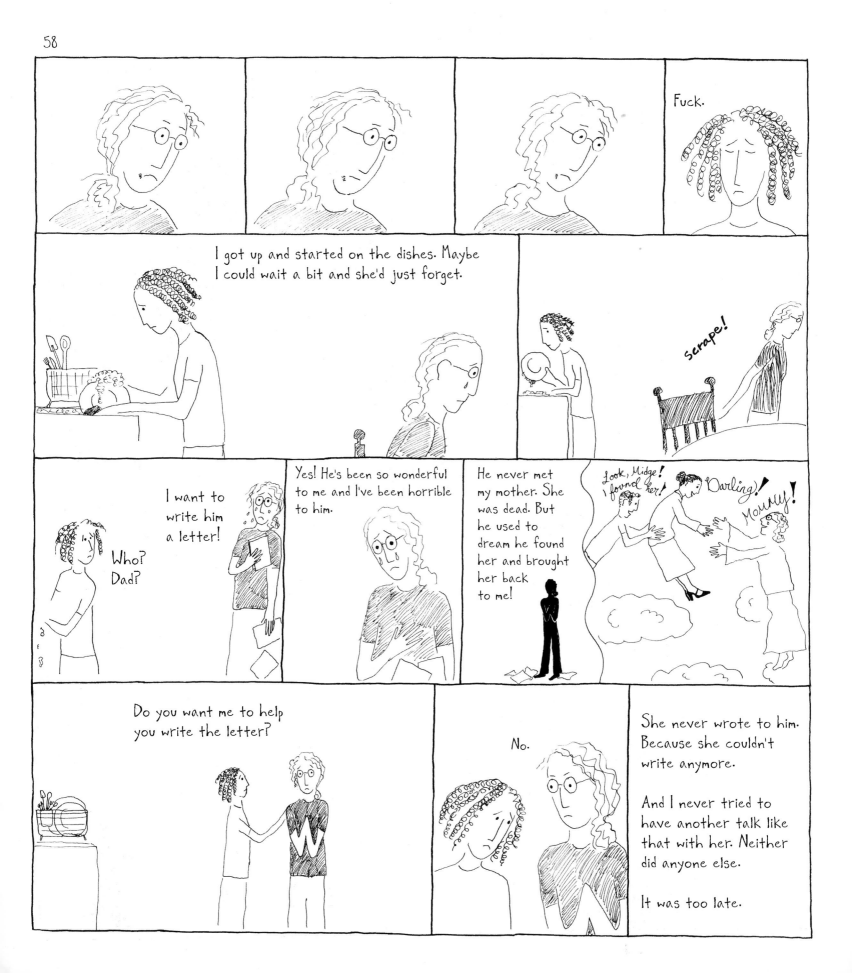

One of the first things that happened to Mom when she got sick was that she lost her sense of smell. This can be a sign of Alzheimer's. But that was before we even suspected that she had something serious. She just couldn't smell.

Of course later we realized: it was one of the first steps in her separation from the world.

It frightened her.

She could not smell garlic or apples or tomatoes that had warmed in the summer sun.

Mom had never let us have sugar when we were kids.

And she never craved it herself. Unlike me. I gorged on it in secret.

But as her sense of smell diminished, she seemed to discover the pleasure of sweetness on the tongue.

She began to grab at sugar.

She ate as much as she could, even when she couldn't figure out how to unwrap it.

Mom forgot more and more of herself.

She didn't know that she thought sugar was evil. She only knew it tasted good. I used to hide candy so I wouldn't get in trouble. Now I hid it so she wouldn't eat it all.

Mom dressed herself in odd collections of garments from different seasons and occasions.

Guatemalan hat almost always

accessories and footwear carried around until abandoned

← messy hair

← turtleneck even when hot

dressy office skirt

socks   undies

shirts

sweaters

Sometimes she realized what she was doing partway through.

Maybe I could start a new style!

Mom wore winter clothes that summer, so she sweated a lot.

And she didn't brush her teeth very well, so her breath stank.

I was so embarrassed. It reminded me of when I was a teenager and I wouldn't walk with her at the mall because she dressed weird.

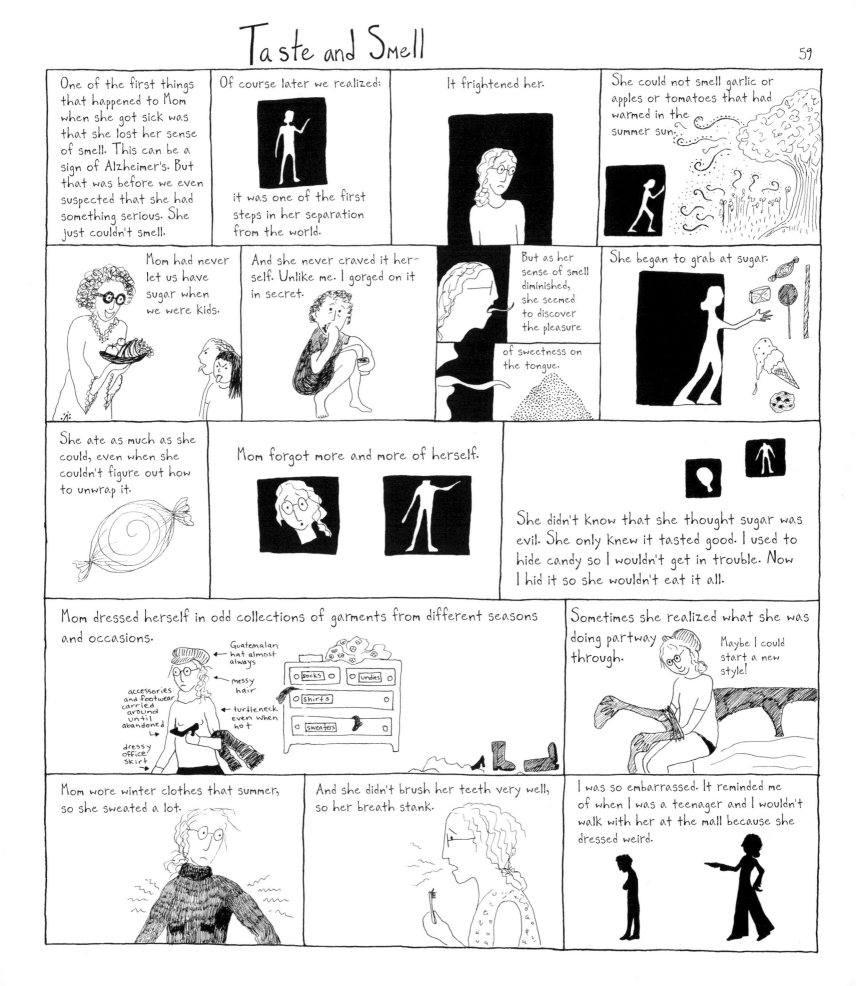

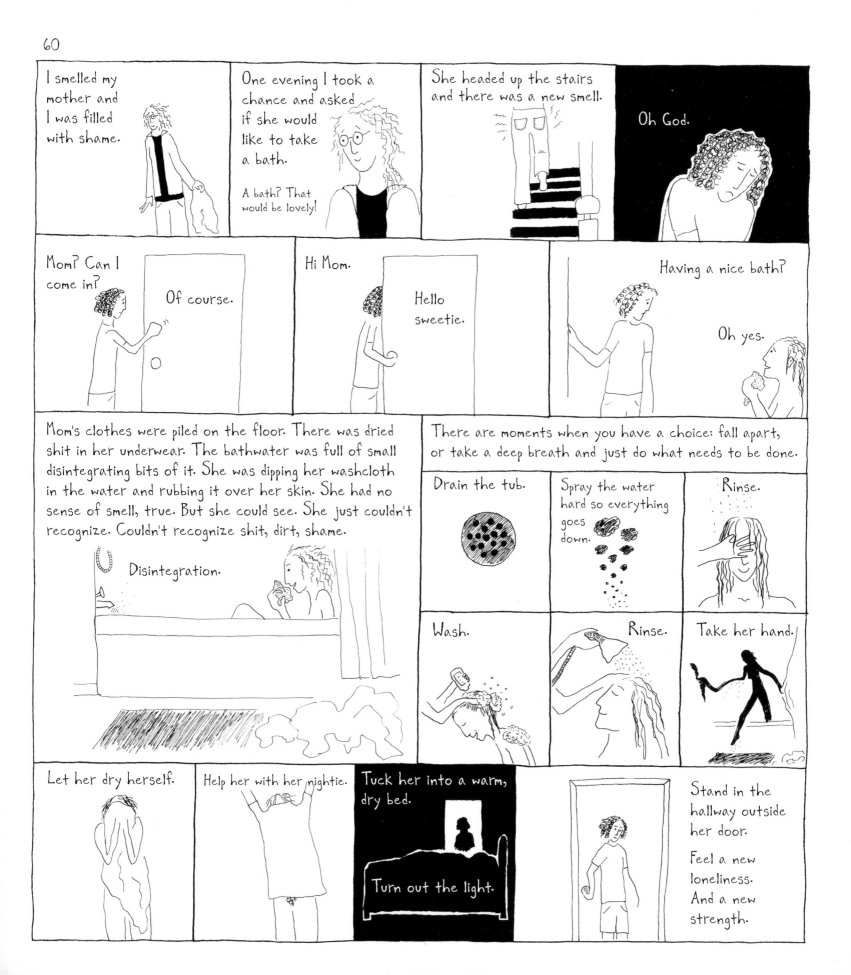

I smelled my mother and I was filled with shame.

One evening I took a chance and asked if she would like to take a bath.

A bath? That would be lovely!

She headed up the stairs and there was a new smell.

Oh God.

Mom? Can I come in?

Of course.

Hi Mom.

Hello sweetie.

Having a nice bath?

Oh yes.

Mom's clothes were piled on the floor. There was dried shit in her underwear. The bathwater was full of small disintegrating bits of it. She was dipping her washcloth in the water and rubbing it over her skin. She had no sense of smell, true. But she could see. She just couldn't recognize. Couldn't recognize shit, dirt, shame.

Disintegration.

There are moments when you have a choice: fall apart, or take a deep breath and just do what needs to be done.

Drain the tub.

Spray the water hard so everything goes down.

Rinse.

Wash.

Rinse.

Take her hand.

Let her dry herself.

Help her with her nightie.

Tuck her into a warm, dry bed.

Turn out the light.

Stand in the hallway outside her door.

Feel a new loneliness. And a new strength.

Me: Bathroom stuff seems harder for you lately.

Mom: Oy.

Me: Yeah...

Mom: Harder... that's not fair is it?

Me: No, none of it's fair at all, Mom.

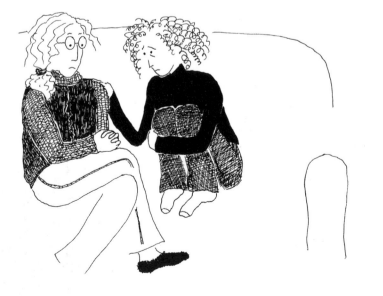

Trouble Understanding

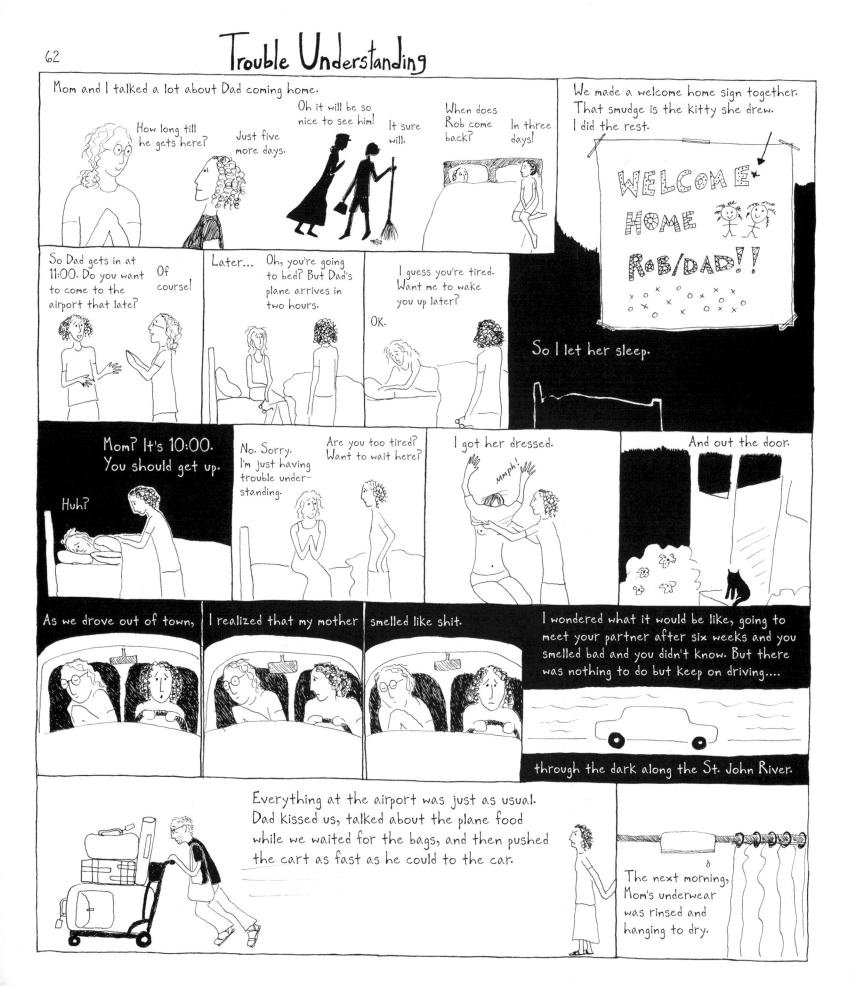

Hair

Most people in my family have curly hair. It was one of the things that made us really stand out in the small towns we lived in when I was growing up.

Mom had tried to straighten her hair for a while in the 60s. She ironed it.

She rolled it tightly around large juice cans.

ow.

She and Dad both tried a thick, waxy product meant for black people's hair. It stuck in their hair for months.

In the late 70s, Mom got her hair cut in a short, round afro-ish style. When she came home, I told her she looked "perfectly hideous." I like to think I was just trying out new vocabulary.

From about the mid 80s on, Mom wore her hair the same way: long, pulled back in a ponytail, usually a little fuzzy.

My friends' moms had tight perms. They also wore a lot of makeup.

I saw your mother the other day, Sarah. I could tell it was her, even from the back. No one else wears their hair like that! Bless her heart.

When I was little, Mom had to fight with me to brush the knots out of my hair. She wrote me a story with pictures about me running away to escape the hairbrush. It was called Sarah and the Monster. In the story I hide in a tunnel and meet a monster.

The monster goes and takes my place at home because she actually wants her hair brushed.

After a few weeks or months I give up and come out of the tunnel. When Mom sees me, we run towards each other so fast that there is a huge bump when we meet. We kiss and hug and jump up and down and twirl around and around.

Then I let her brush my hair and only scream and bite a little bit because I am so glad to be home again with my mom.

This is the kind of thing I would think about whenever I washed or untangled my mom's hair when she was sick.

I never used a comb or brush on Mom's hair, just my fingers. At some point I started putting little balls of her hair in my pocket instead of throwing them away.

And then I started collecting my own hair. Every time I washed my hair or ran my fingers through it, I kept the loose hairs. It did not take long to collect boxes of dense, springy clumps of hair.

January - Sept 2000

Some of my friends found it disturbing.

Eek!

I found it comforting. I collected more and more and more.

Sept 01 - Mar 02

April - Aug 2001

I kept the boxes on shelves above the bed and it helped me sleep at night, just knowing they were there.

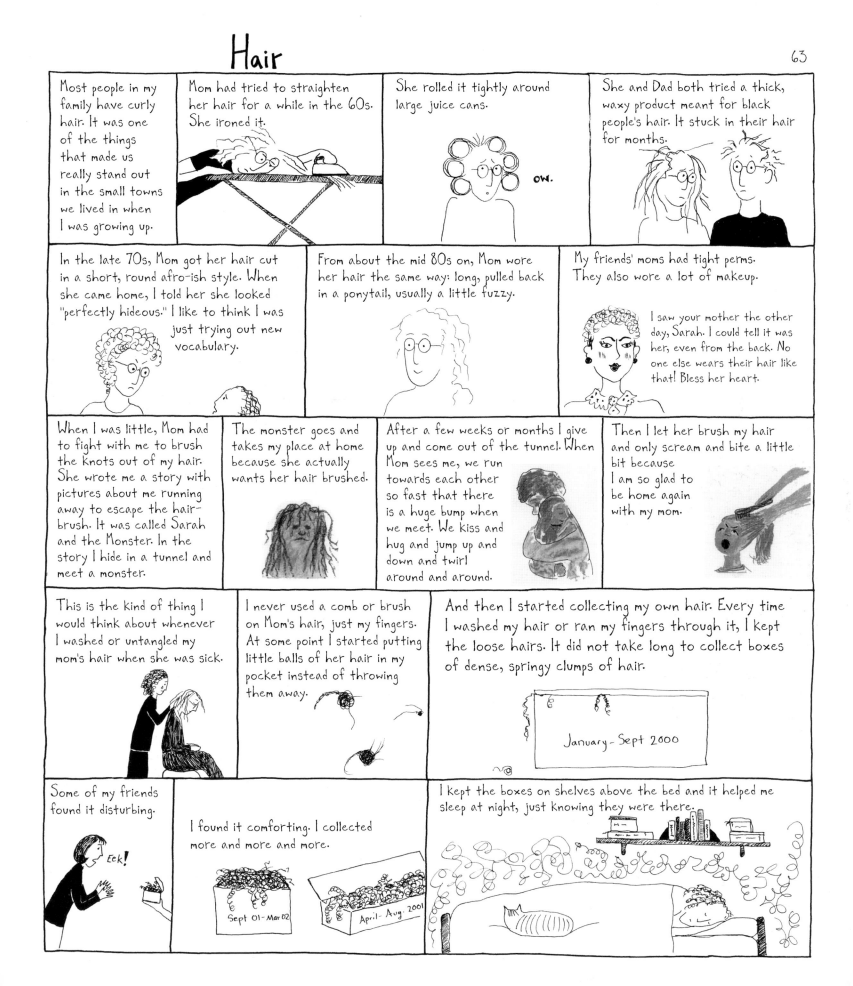

A Small Joke

We were listening to Bob Marley, but I can't remember
which song. Probably One Foundation or Positive Vibration.

Did he say constipation?
Oh, excuse me!

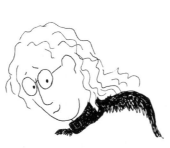

Kitty, The

My parents used to have a cat that everyone called The Kitty. She was even addressed that way, as in "Hello, The Kitty," or "Come here, The Kitty."

Mom had named her Lucy when they first got her, and it pissed her off when we called her The Kitty. But we couldn't help it.

The summer that Mom started getting sick, The Kitty stopped eating and drinking.

The vet came to the house and put her to sleep while Mom held her.

Ready, Midge?

They buried her in the garden and planted a miniature rosebush on her grave.

They spent a year in mourning.

The next summer they got another black cat from the SPCA. We all had trouble remembering the former cat; the two blended together into one continuous female black cat.

Mom named this one Lucy, too, and we tried harder this time to call her by that name.

But it was still a challenge.

Hi The Kit... I mean, Lucy.

Lucy was stocky, with small ears and round, close-set eyes.

She looked like the offspring of the Owl and the Pussycat.

Mom loved all animals. But she was obsessed with Lucy.

There you are, darling!

Oh! Look how smart she is!

Beautiful!

Just look at her eating her food!

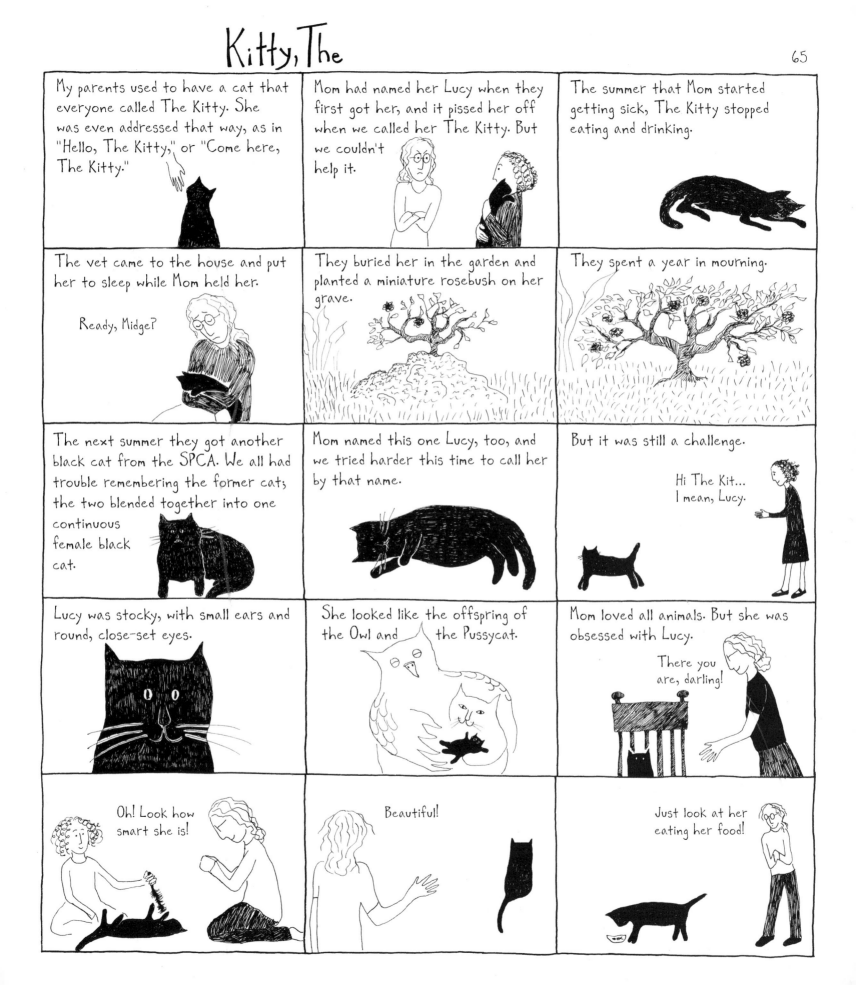

Lucy never seemed to care about people that much.

She spent a good part of the day under the covers on Mom and Dad's bed.

Or under the shed.

Or in the tall grass near the garden.

According to Mom, Lucy was very affectionate.

But not long after they got Lucy, Mom's movements got too unpredictable for any cat, especially an aloof one.

Lucy! Come here, darling, so I can brush you!

Lucy only cuddled with Dad. She sat on his lap occasionally, and he would rest his coffee cup on her flat head. She seemed to like it.

After a brief period of sleeping on my parents' bed at night, Lucy didn't come near Mom much at all. But Mom never seemed to realize this.

She would always ask where Lucy was when she went to bed. At some point we started lying and saying that Lucy was in the room. It helped her calm down and go to sleep.

Sometimes Mom's undying love for Lucy drove me crazy. It pissed me off that she couldn't see what Lucy was really like.

Kitty kitty KITTY kitty! Kitty KITTY kitty kitty Kitty KITTY kitty Kitty

Lucy! You don't know how good you have it here, ungrateful cat!

I sometimes got a small, mean satisfaction from speaking the unspeakable.

She's the coldest cat I've ever met!

Huh?

Shh!

But then I would relent.

Wow, Mom, look how great Lucy is!

Yeah!

I made Mom little books about Lucy, and cards and small photo albums. She liked to carry them around.

Queen Lucy by Sarah

Happy Mother's Day!

PHOTOS OF LUCY for MOM

She recognized and talked about Lucy even when she seemed confused about who I was.

Is it weird to be jealous of a cat?

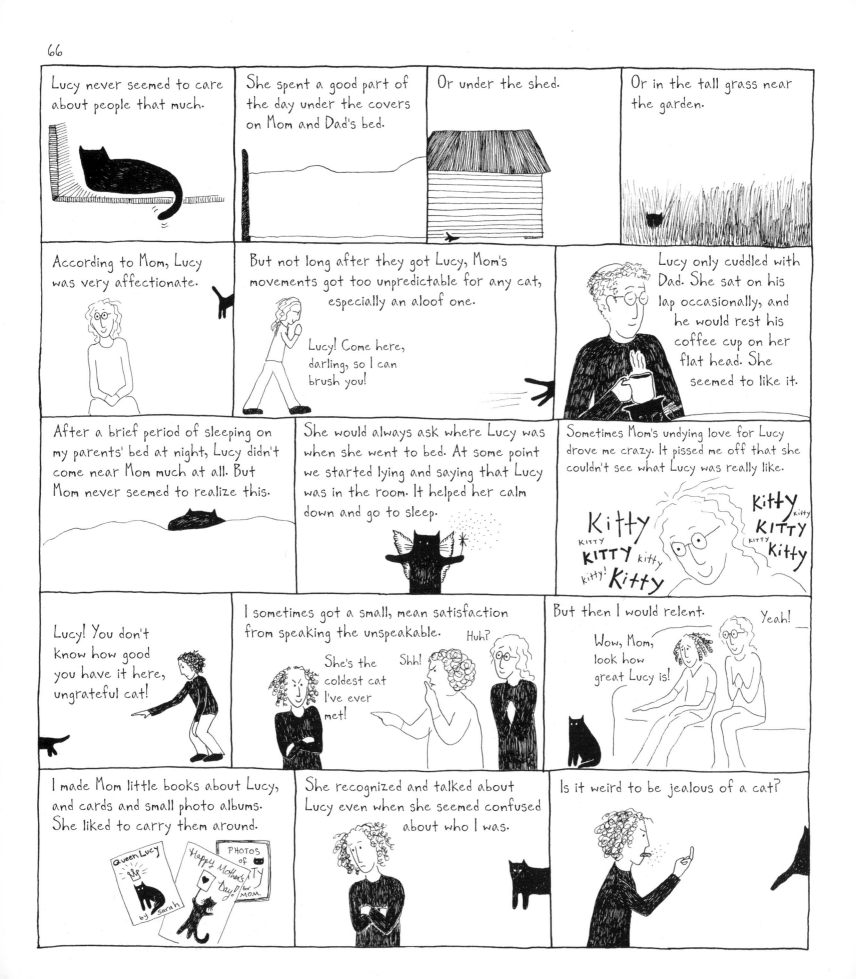

One Sunday morning a close friend of mine called to tell me that her grandmother had killed herself.

They found her in her car in the closed carport with the engine running.

She had left a medical book on her coffee table.

I had met her once. She was a wealthy, elegant old lady.

It was open to the chapter on Alzheimer's.

The same day I heard about this, Mom and Dad called for our usual Sunday chat.

When I asked Mom how she was, she told Dad to go outside so she could talk to me privately.

I don't want to be married anymore!

Shit. Mom had never talked to me about marriage problems or anything like that. I was her kid, not her confidante.

I'M a NOBODY!

I'm not a REAL PERSON anymore!

Then she started crying really hard. I decided to pretend she wasn't my mother so I could manage to stay on the phone and listen to her.

Mmm hmm. Oh it must be so hard.

Yes I'm sure you do.

And how do you feel about that?

She said Dad was treating her like a child. She wanted to live by herself. She wanted to be left alone. We talked for an hour or so. Then...

OK. So you're going to sit down with Dad and tell him how you feel? Promise? Great.

Click.

WAAAH! I want my MOMMY!

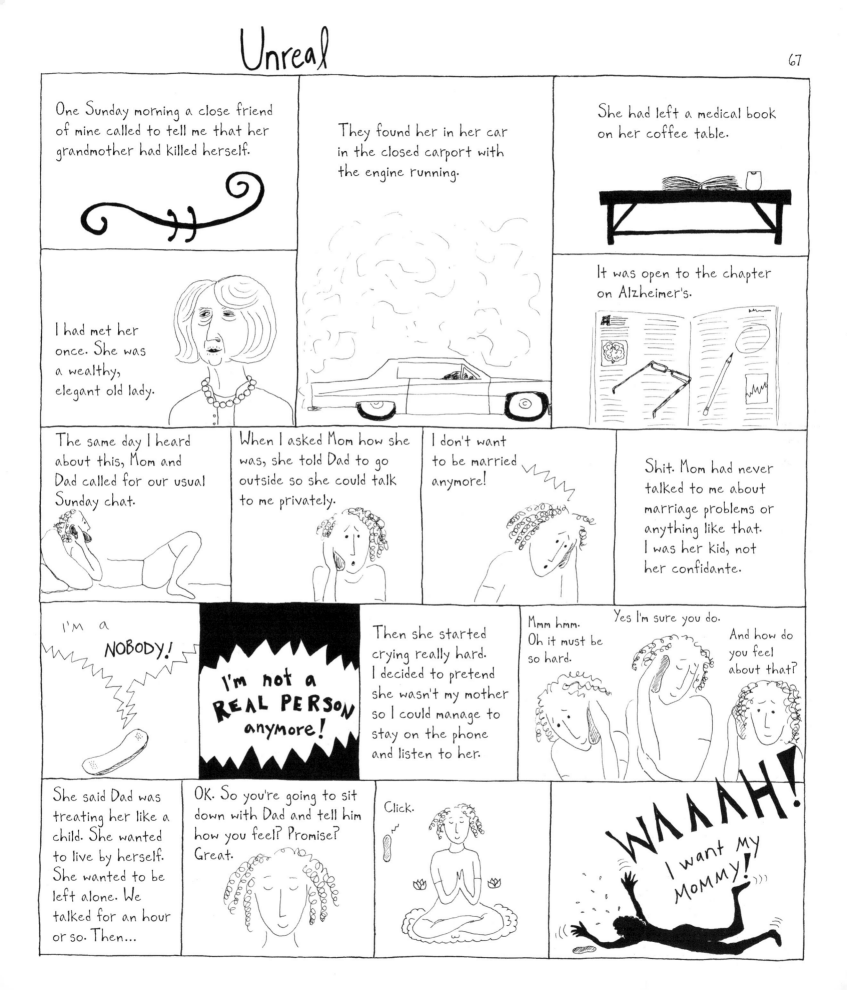

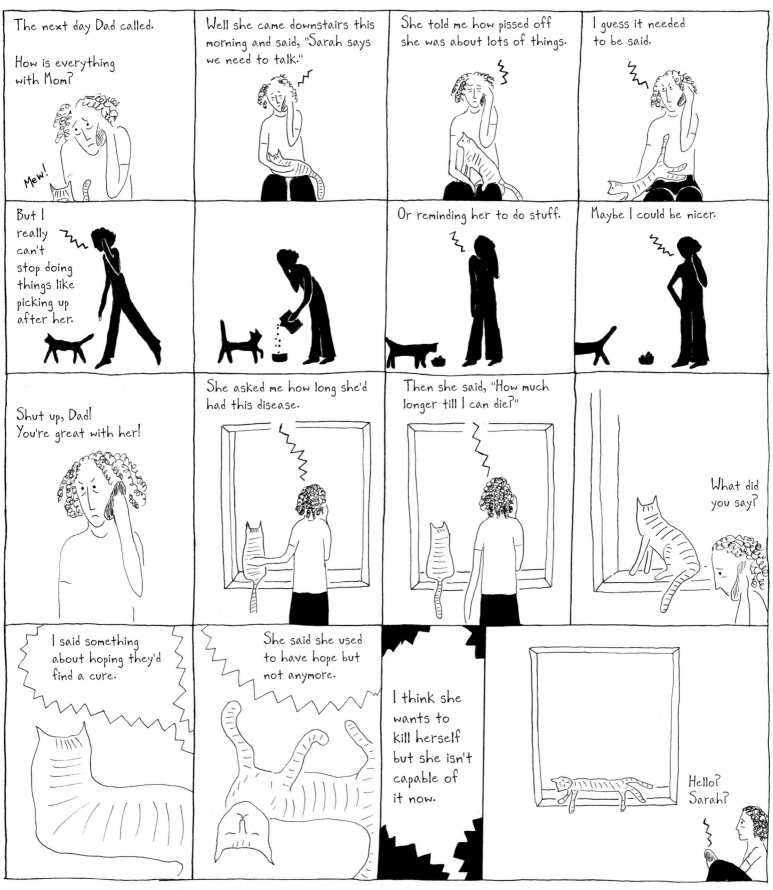

Love to Donimo

Hope you like Bmbows.
See you soon   The whole
family is
            ears to see you
            from Midge

Gaps

I spent the next summer writing left-handed to strengthen my brain.
I filled pages and pages with alphabets and encouraging notes to myself.

ABCDEFGHIJKLMNOPQRSTUVWXYZ
abcdefghijklmnopqrstuvwxyz sarah → getting better!

When I visited Mom, I wrote left-handed every night in one journal and kept my sketches and notes in another.

URGENT!

She points to things— sometimes in the wrong direction or at the wrong thing. She wiggles her index finger at things or at you when she can't think of the right word and she wants you to know what she means...

She wiggles her finger, then sees her finger wiggling and wiggles the finger on her other hand, then rubs that finger all over her other hand. Why?

Mom did not know what "tank top" meant.

She didn't recognize pineapple weed, which we always called chamomile, and which we used to pick and eat together when I was a kid.

matricaria discoidea

One day we took a walk and we passed a preteen boy on the street.

Oh! That was Jessica. How nice of her to remember us!

One morning she stood behind me grinding her teeth as I tried to eat some eggs.

CRUNCH! CRUNCH!

I have good news for you and Hannah. Things are getting better. Lots of research.

I knew what she meant. Research for a cure for Alzheimer's. I lost my appetite.

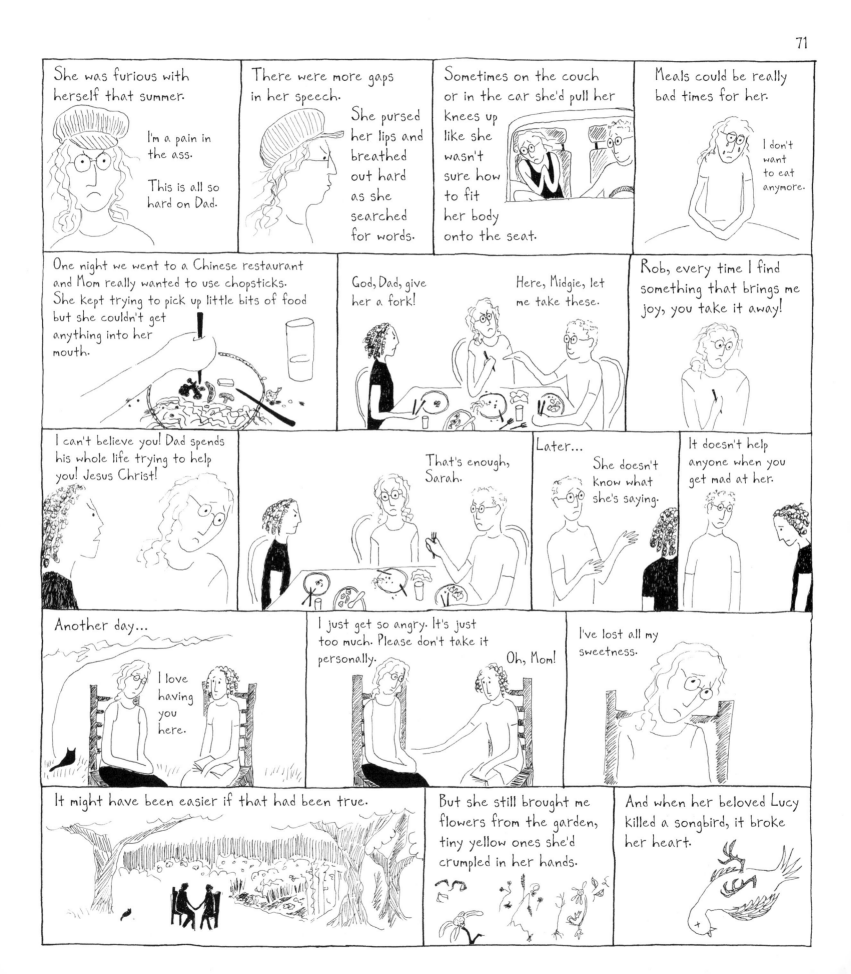

She was furious with herself that summer.

I'm a pain in the ass.

This is all so hard on Dad.

There were more gaps in her speech.

She pursed her lips and breathed out hard as she searched for words.

Sometimes on the couch or in the car she'd pull her knees up like she wasn't sure how to fit her body onto the seat.

Meals could be really bad times for her.

I don't want to eat anymore.

One night we went to a Chinese restaurant and Mom really wanted to use chopsticks. She kept trying to pick up little bits of food but she couldn't get anything into her mouth.

God, Dad, give her a fork!

Here, Midgie, let me take these.

Rob, every time I find something that brings me joy, you take it away!

I can't believe you! Dad spends his whole life trying to help you! Jesus Christ!

That's enough, Sarah.

Later...

She doesn't know what she's saying.

It doesn't help anyone when you get mad at her.

Another day...

I love having you here.

I just get so angry. It's just too much. Please don't take it personally.

Oh, Mom!

I've lost all my sweetness.

It might have been easier if that had been true.

But she still brought me flowers from the garden, tiny yellow ones she'd crumpled in her hands.

And when her beloved Lucy killed a songbird, it broke her heart.

One day we were all sitting around talking
about not remembering books or movies and
watching them again and realizing we'd already
seen them. Mom said ruefully, "Every day is like
that for me. I get up and I think it's a new
early morning and Rob says no, it's 11 PM."

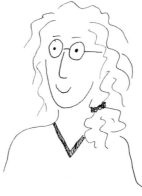

Bird Brain

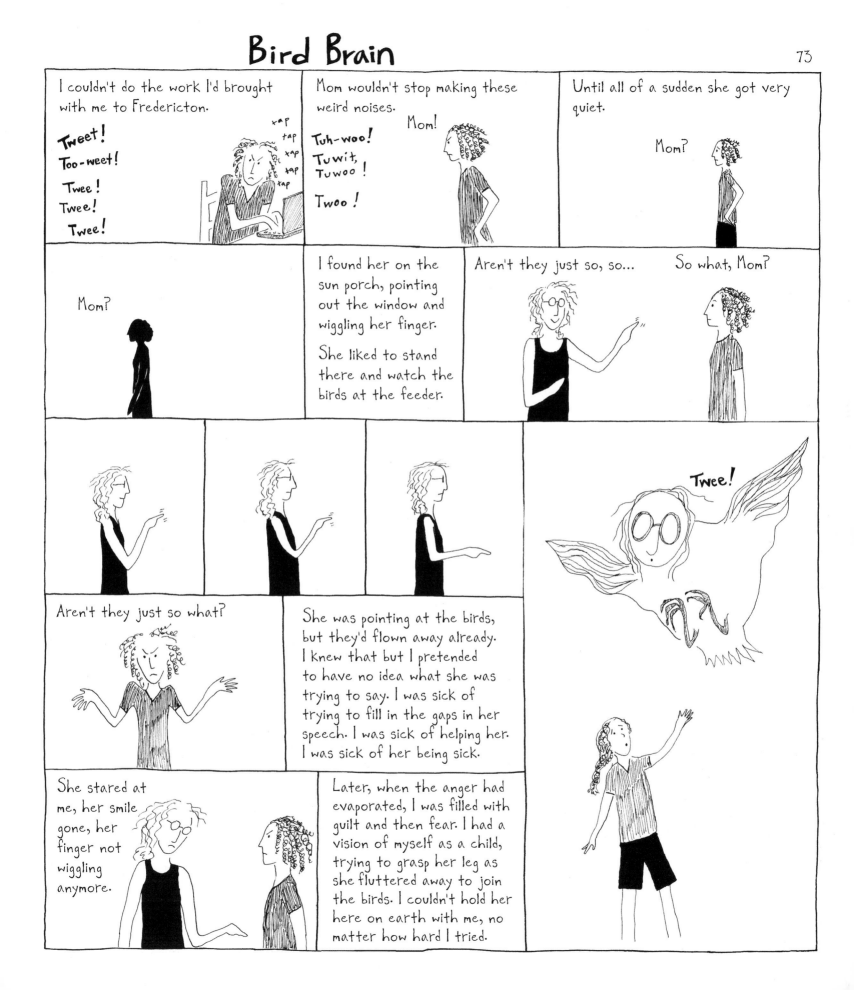

I Wasn't There

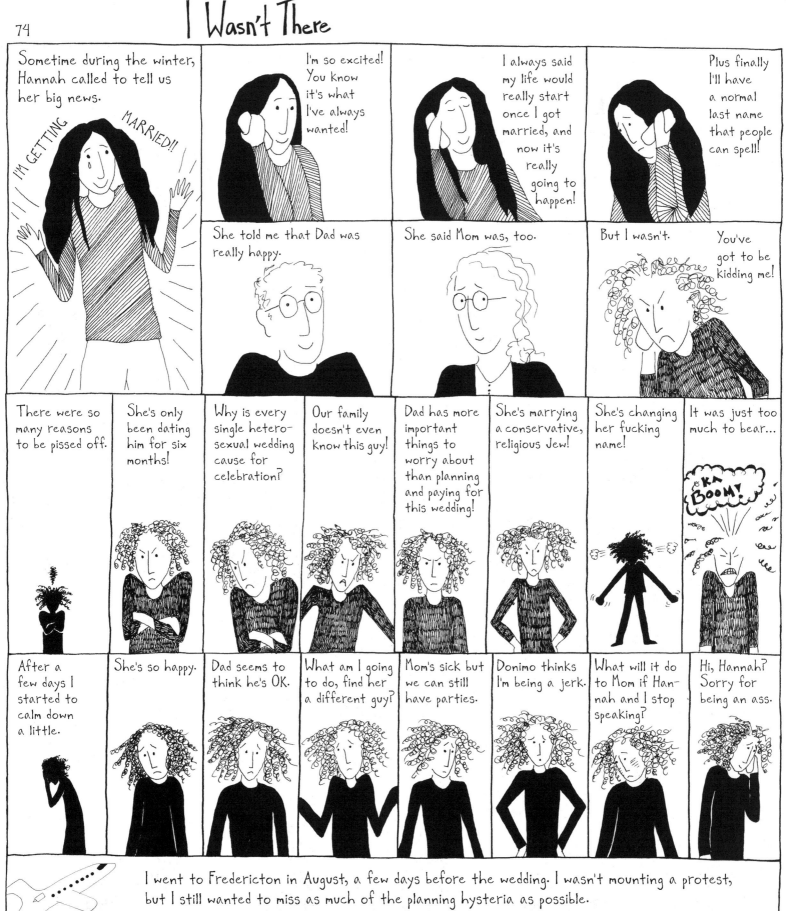

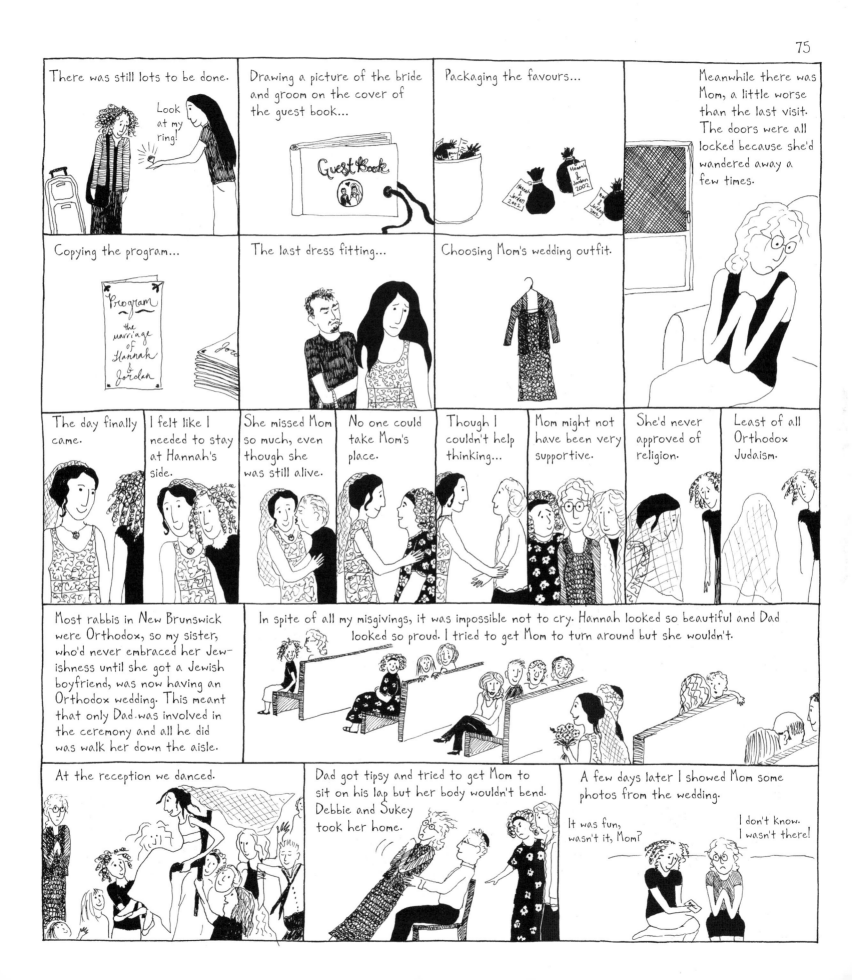

There was still lots to be done.

Look at my ring!

Drawing a picture of the bride and groom on the cover of the guest book...

Guest Book

Packaging the favours...

Meanwhile there was Mom, a little worse than the last visit. The doors were all locked because she'd wandered away a few times.

Copying the program...

Program
the marriage of Hannah & Jordan

The last dress fitting...

Choosing Mom's wedding outfit.

The day finally came.

I felt like I needed to stay at Hannah's side.

She missed Mom so much, even though she was still alive.

No one could take Mom's place.

Though I couldn't help thinking...

Mom might not have been very supportive.

She'd never approved of religion.

Least of all Orthodox Judaism.

Most rabbis in New Brunswick were Orthodox, so my sister, who'd never embraced her Jewishness until she got a Jewish boyfriend, was now having an Orthodox wedding. This meant that only Dad was involved in the ceremony and all he did was walk her down the aisle.

In spite of all my misgivings, it was impossible not to cry. Hannah looked so beautiful and Dad looked so proud. I tried to get Mom to turn around but she wouldn't.

At the reception we danced.

Dad got tipsy and tried to get Mom to sit on his lap but her body wouldn't bend. Debbie and Sukey took her home.

A few days later I showed Mom some photos from the wedding.

It was fun, wasn't it, Mom?

I don't know. I wasn't there!

Water

I choked on some food and started drinking water from my glass.

Mom: Are you OK? Why don't you have some water?

Me: I am, I'm drinking water right now.

Mom: I mean for your coughing.

Mom: Ooh, I would love lots and lots of water.

[Drinks three small glasses.]

See how happy she was with all that water?

Finally

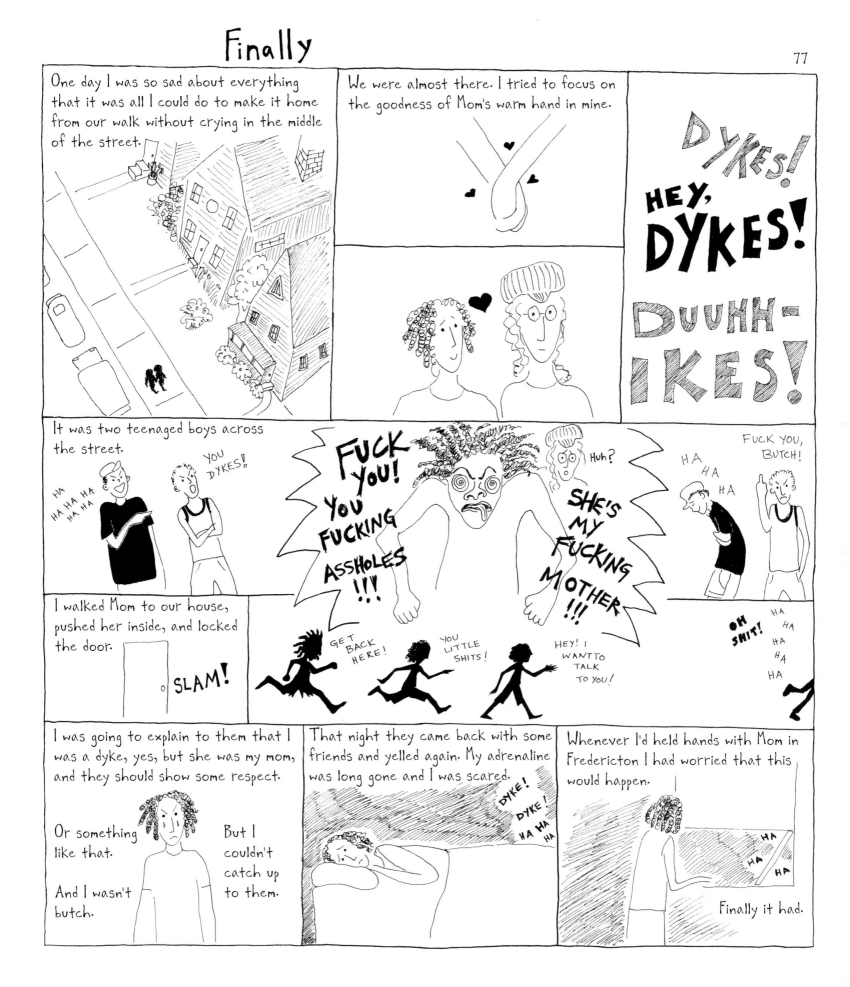

One day I was so sad about everything that it was all I could do to make it home from our walk without crying in the middle of the street.

We were almost there. I tried to focus on the goodness of Mom's warm hand in mine.

DYKES! HEY, DYKES! DUUHH-IKES!

It was two teenaged boys across the street.

HA HA HA HA HA HA

YOU DYKES!!

FUCK YOU! YOU FUCKING ASSHOLES!!!...

Huh?

SHE'S MY FUCKING MOTHER!!!

HA HA HA

FUCK YOU, BUTCH!

I walked Mom to our house, pushed her inside, and locked the door.

SLAM!

GET BACK HERE!

YOU LITTLE SHITS!

HEY! I WANT TO TALK TO YOU!

OH SHIT!

HA HA HA HA HA

I was going to explain to them that I was a dyke, yes, but she was my mom, and they should show some respect.

Or something like that.

And I wasn't butch.

But I couldn't catch up to them.

That night they came back with some friends and yelled again. My adrenaline was long gone and I was scared.

DYKE! DYKE! HA HA HA

Whenever I'd held hands with Mom in Fredericton I had worried that this would happen.

HA HA HA

Finally it had.

Thunderstorm

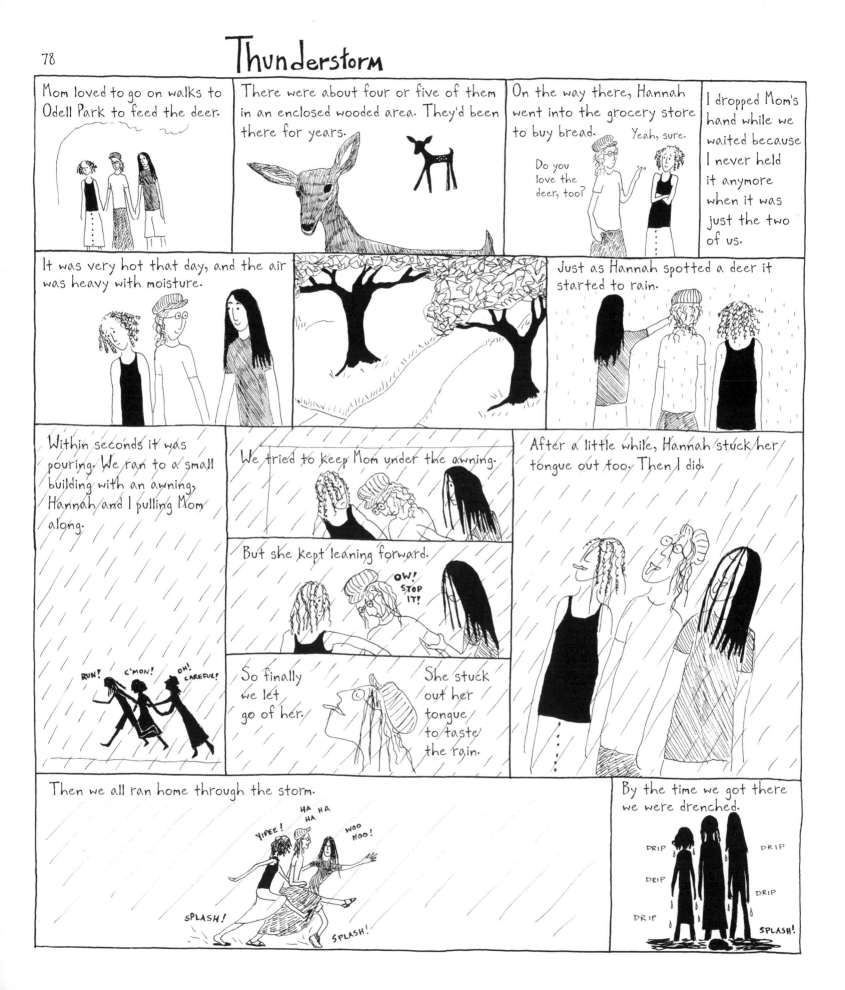

Mom started running ahead of us.
She looked so normal when she ran.
For some reason she looked more
coordinated.

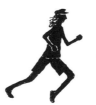

Run Away!

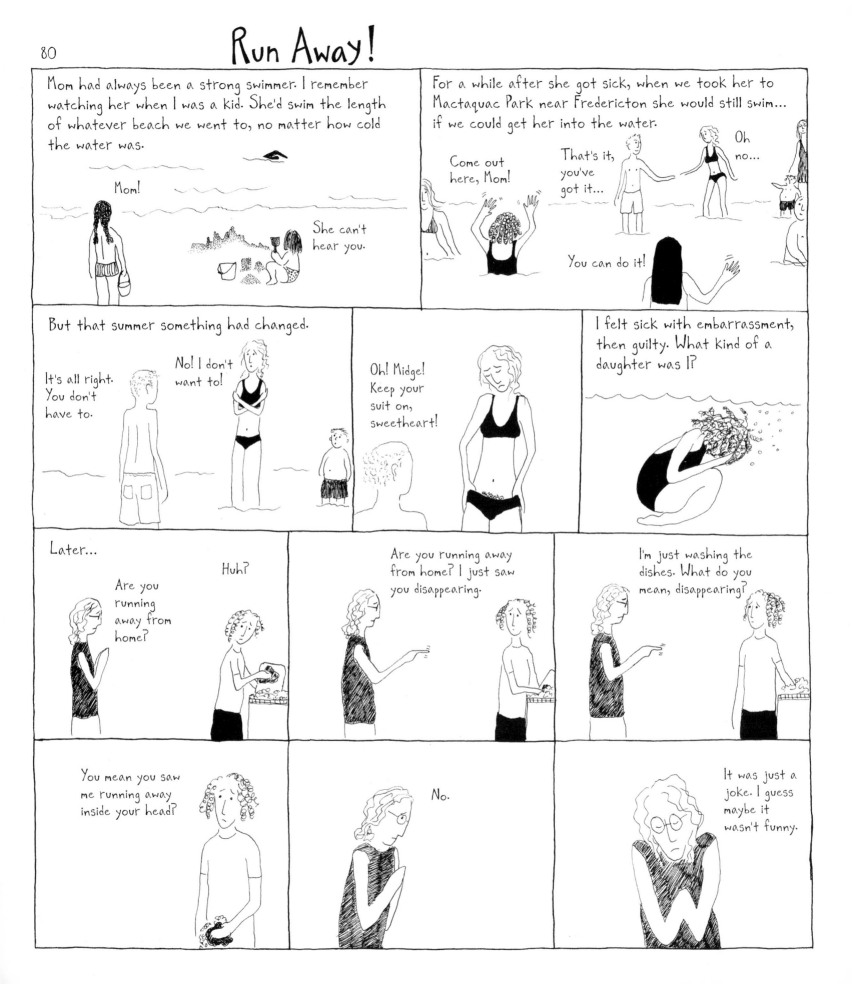

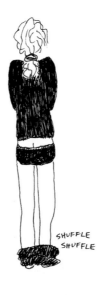

Mom came out of the bathroom and started wandering off down the hall. "I feel left out," she murmured to herself.

SHUFFLE
SHUFFLE

How's it going, Mom?

Oh, I think it's going
quite sadly.

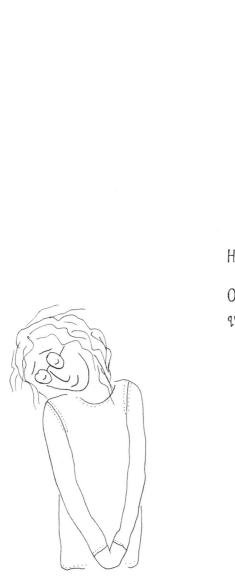

Part Three

Things that Mom liked to carry around

Mom liked to carry things with her when she wandered around the house.
She'd go through phases of carrying the same thing for a while.

> cat brush
> weeds from the garden
> photos of her parents
> greeting cards
> books I made her
> socks
> The Lord of the Rings, Book One: The Fellowship of the Ring
> napkins
> bits of houseplants

Cut My Life Into Pieces

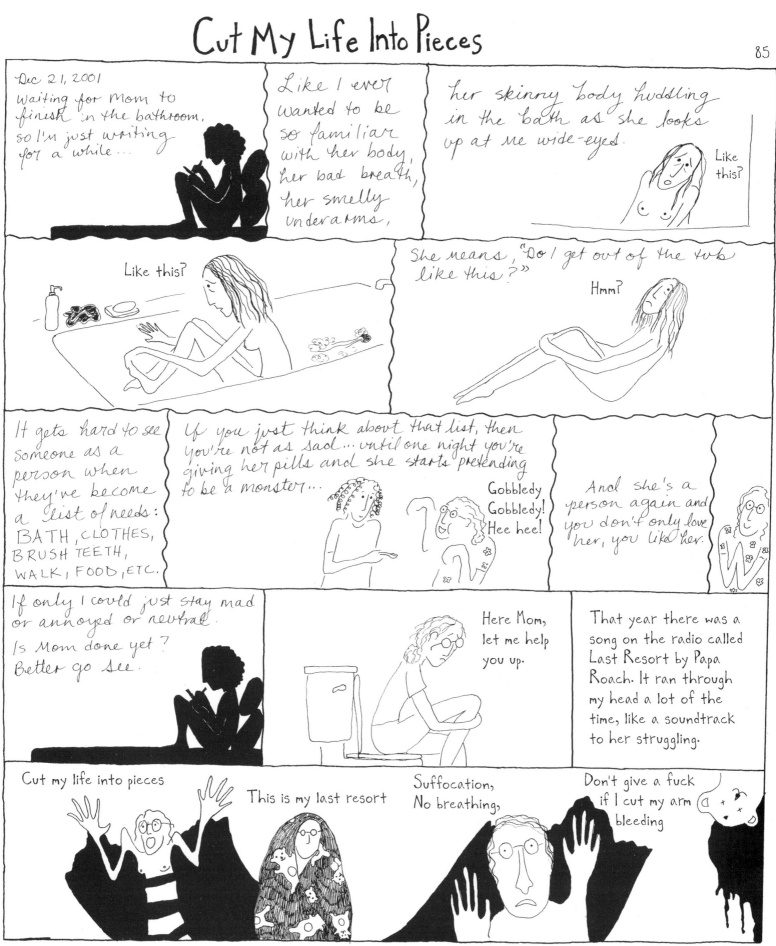

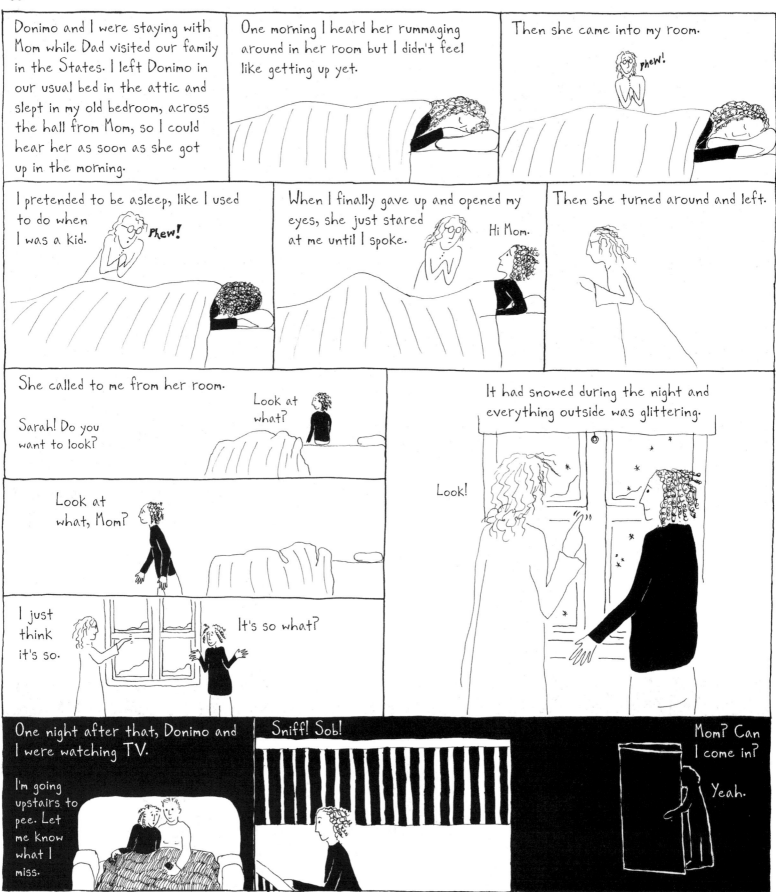

Donimo and I were staying with Mom while Dad visited our family in the States. I left Donimo in our usual bed in the attic and slept in my old bedroom, across the hall from Mom, so I could hear her as soon as she got up in the morning.

One morning I heard her rummaging around in her room but I didn't feel like getting up yet.

Then she came into my room.

phew!

I pretended to be asleep, like I used to do when I was a kid.

Phew!

When I finally gave up and opened my eyes, she just stared at me until I spoke.

Hi Mom.

Then she turned around and left.

She called to me from her room.

Sarah! Do you want to look?

Look at what?

Look at what, Mom?

It had snowed during the night and everything outside was glittering.

Look!

I just think it's so.

It's so what?

One night after that, Donimo and I were watching TV.

I'm going upstairs to pee. Let me know what I miss.

Sniff! Sob!

Mom? Can I come in?

Yeah.

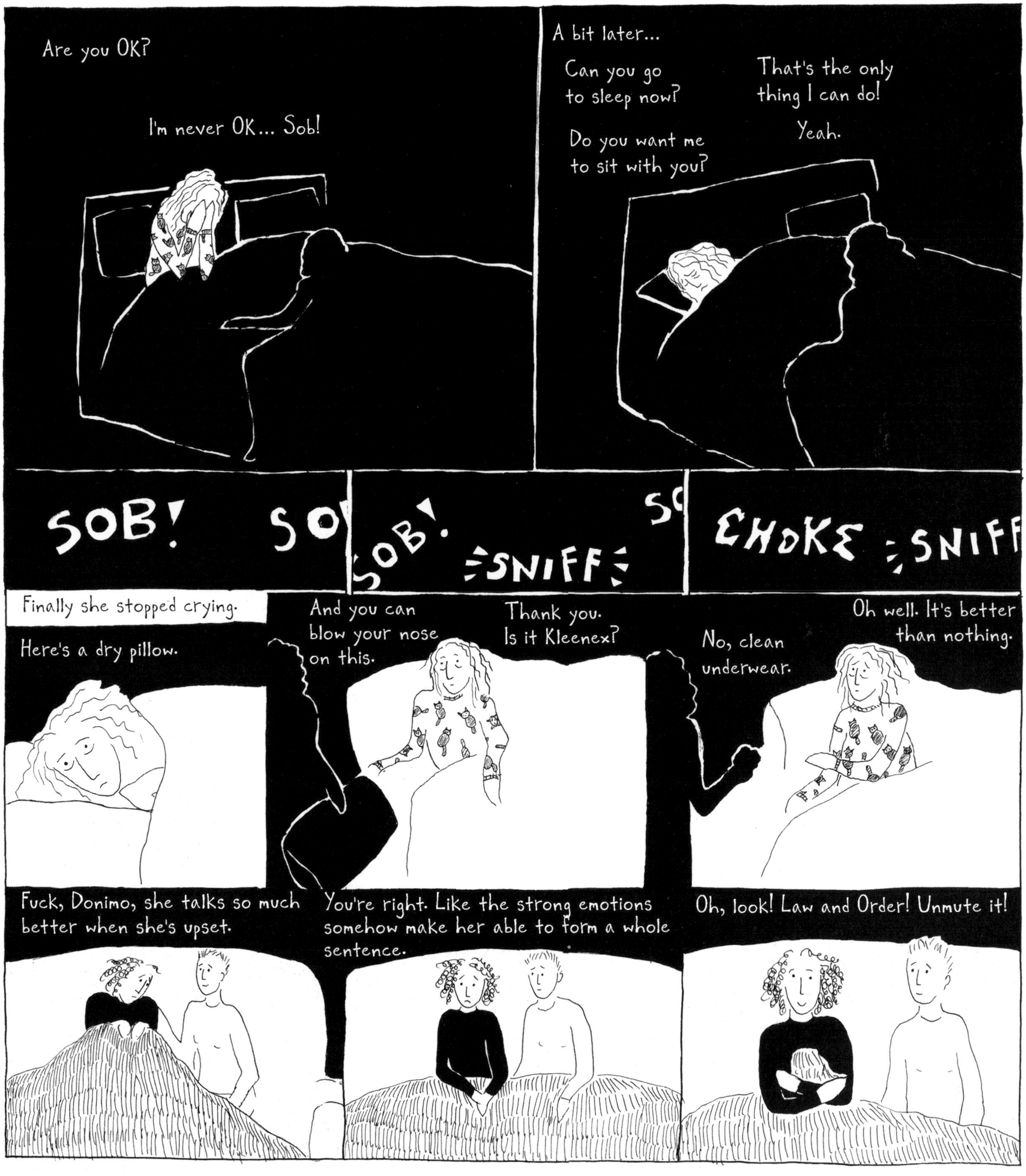
Are you OK?
I'm never OK... Sob!
A bit later...
Can you go to sleep now?
That's the only thing I can do!
Do you want me to sit with you?
Yeah.
SOB!
SO
SOB!
SNIFF
SC
CHOKE
SNIFF
Finally she stopped crying.
Here's a dry pillow.
And you can blow your nose on this.
Thank you. Is it Kleenex?
No, clean underwear.
Oh well. It's better than nothing.
Fuck, Donimo, she talks so much better when she's upset.
You're right. Like the strong emotions somehow make her able to form a whole sentence.
Oh, look! Law and Order! Unmute it!

Questions

Mom: Are you guys guy?
So you don't have to
wonder about.

Me: Are you comfortable, Mom?
Mom: I don't know.

Mom: Am I a stringle?

Me: Are you OK, Mom?
Mom: No. I just can't tell what is and isn't.

Mom: Honey, can I open
your voice?

Me: Oh, Mom, I thought you were sleeping.
Mom: I don't know if I am or not.

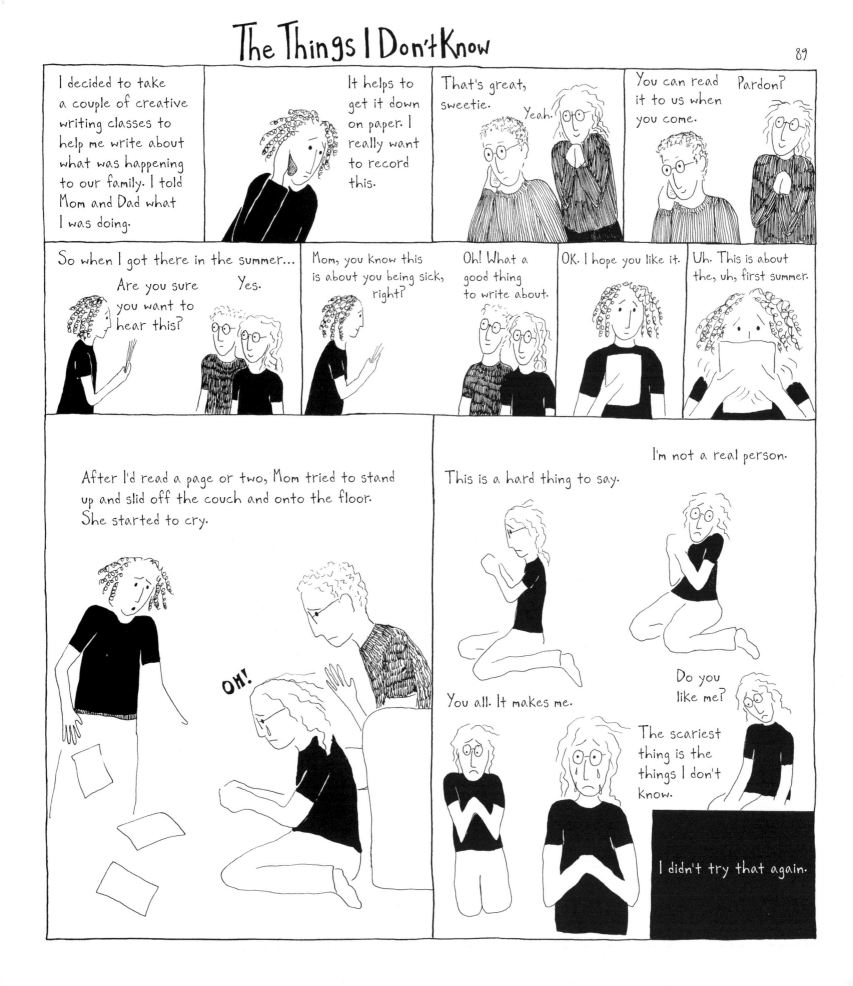

Y Tu Loquita

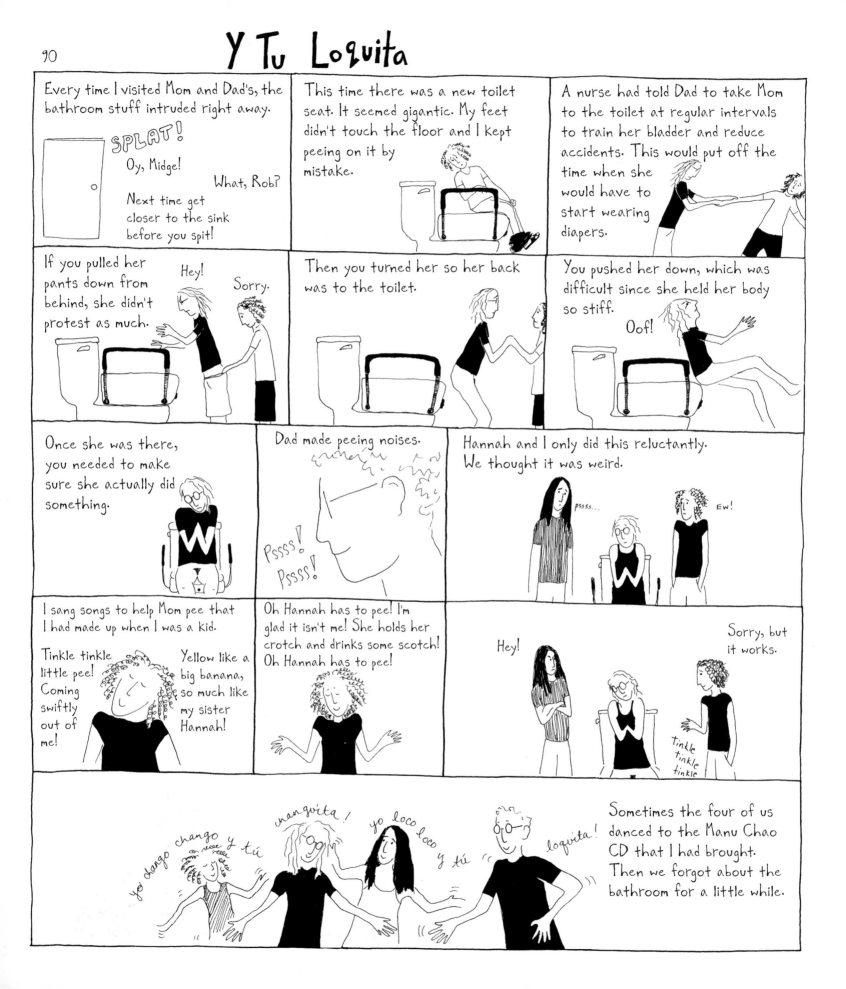

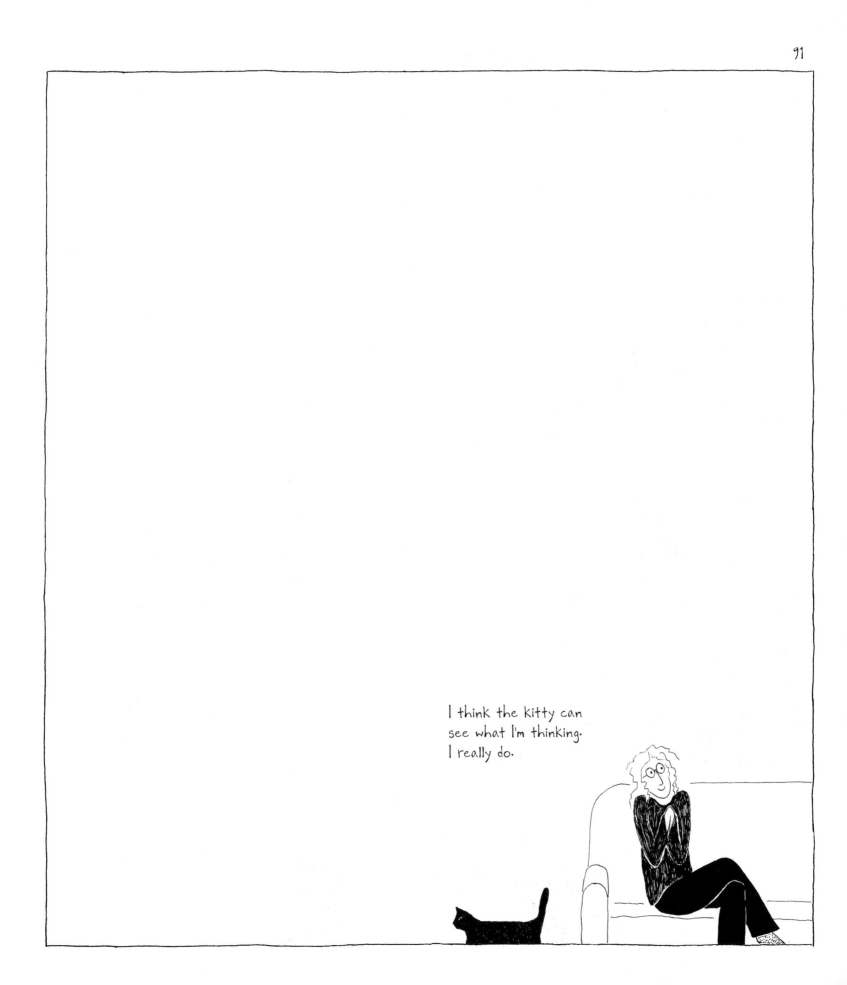

I think the kitty can
see what I'm thinking.
I really do.

Outsiders

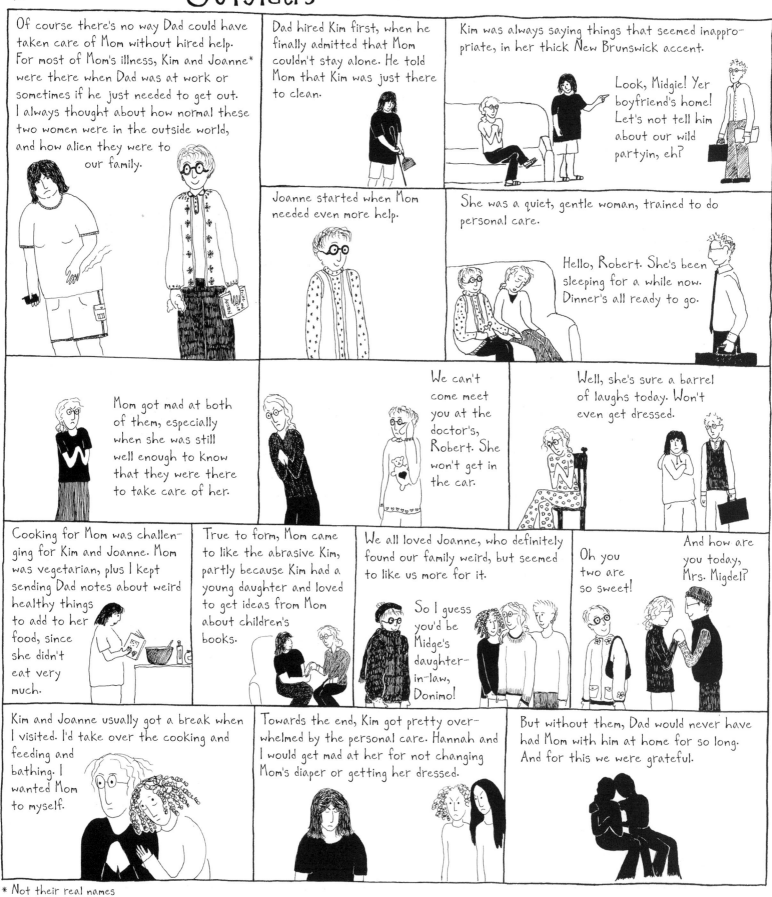

Of course there's no way Dad could have taken care of Mom without hired help. For most of Mom's illness, Kim and Joanne* were there when Dad was at work or sometimes if he just needed to get out. I always thought about how normal these two women were in the outside world, and how alien they were to our family.

Dad hired Kim first, when he finally admitted that Mom couldn't stay alone. He told Mom that Kim was just there to clean.

Kim was always saying things that seemed inappropriate, in her thick New Brunswick accent.

Look, Midgie! Yer boyfriend's home! Let's not tell him about our wild partyin, eh?

Joanne started when Mom needed even more help.

She was a quiet, gentle woman, trained to do personal care.

Hello, Robert. She's been sleeping for a while now. Dinner's all ready to go.

Mom got mad at both of them, especially when she was still well enough to know that they were there to take care of her.

We can't come meet you at the doctor's, Robert. She won't get in the car.

Well, she's sure a barrel of laughs today. Won't even get dressed.

Cooking for Mom was challenging for Kim and Joanne. Mom was vegetarian, plus I kept sending Dad notes about weird healthy things to add to her food, since she didn't eat very much.

True to form, Mom came to like the abrasive Kim, partly because Kim had a young daughter and loved to get ideas from Mom about children's books.

We all loved Joanne, who definitely found our family weird, but seemed to like us more for it.

So I guess you'd be Midge's daughter-in-law, Donimo!

Oh you two are so sweet!

And how are you today, Mrs. Migdel?

Kim and Joanne usually got a break when I visited. I'd take over the cooking and feeding and bathing. I wanted Mom to myself.

Towards the end, Kim got pretty overwhelmed by the personal care. Hannah and I would get mad at her for not changing Mom's diaper or getting her dressed.

But without them, Dad would never have had Mom with him at home for so long. And for this we were grateful.

* Not their real names

Nature Lover

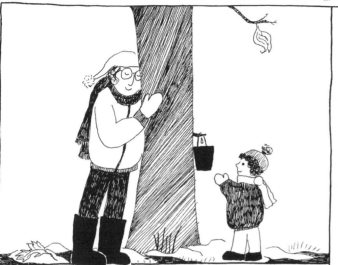

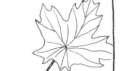

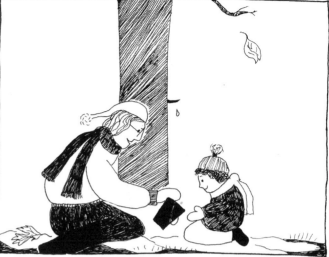

This tree had sweeter sap than the others. We would drink it fresh out of the bucket. We called it "tree juice." It had little bits of bark floating in it.

My mother used to say that she wanted her ashes spread under the sugar maple tree beside the old farmhouse where we lived in Maine.

She also used to say that she wanted to be reincarnated as a maple tree. She felt a strong Kinship with trees, especially maples.

It's hard to make sense of the different things she said. Because she didn't really believe in reincarnation. She always said that death was final. This scared me when I was a kid, thinking that someday I would just end. Then she and Dad pointed out that the idea of living forever was just as incomprehensible and terrifying.

Mom loved all of nature: plants, worms, rocks, soil.

She did not seem to feel as separate from it as most people did.

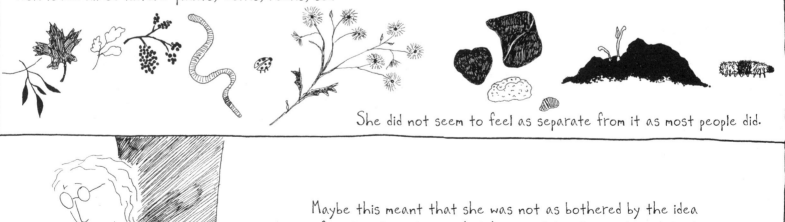

Maybe this meant that she was not as bothered by the idea of just ending; it was what happened to all animals and plants.

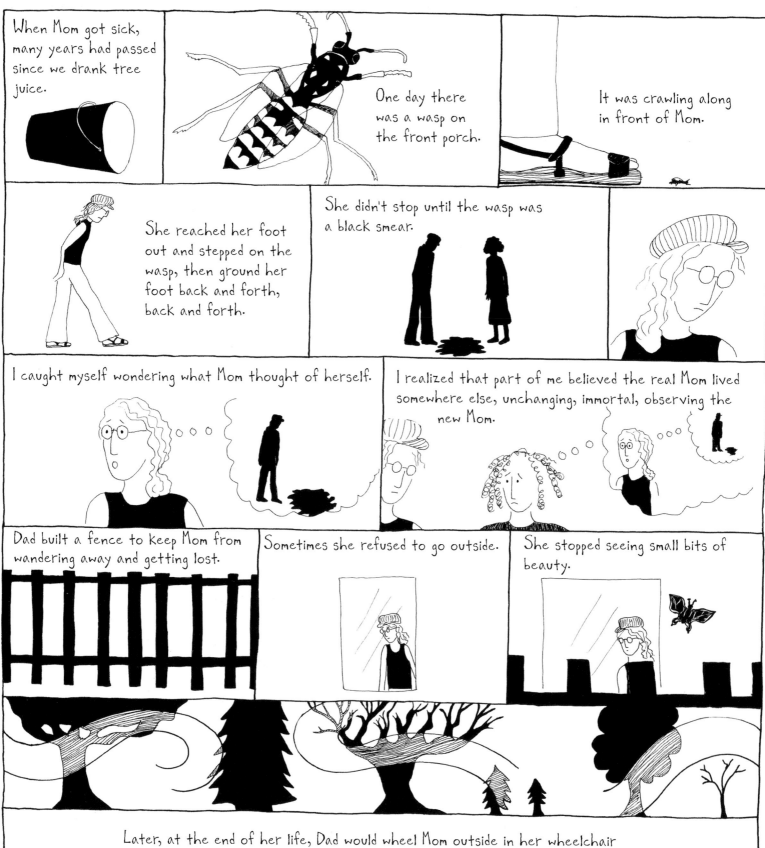

When Mom got sick, many years had passed since we drank tree juice.

One day there was a wasp on the front porch.

It was crawling along in front of Mom.

She reached her foot out and stepped on the wasp, then ground her foot back and forth, back and forth.

She didn't stop until the wasp was a black smear.

I caught myself wondering what Mom thought of herself.

I realized that part of me believed the real Mom lived somewhere else, unchanging, immortal, observing the new Mom.

Dad built a fence to keep Mom from wandering away and getting lost.

Sometimes she refused to go outside.

She stopped seeing small bits of beauty.

Later, at the end of her life, Dad would wheel Mom outside in her wheelchair and they would sit and listen to the wind in the trees. She liked it, he said.

Once I was on the phone with
Mom and I asked her how she was.
"Like this," she said. Then Dad told
me she had spread apart her thumb
and forefinger while she was saying
it, as if to show me what she meant.

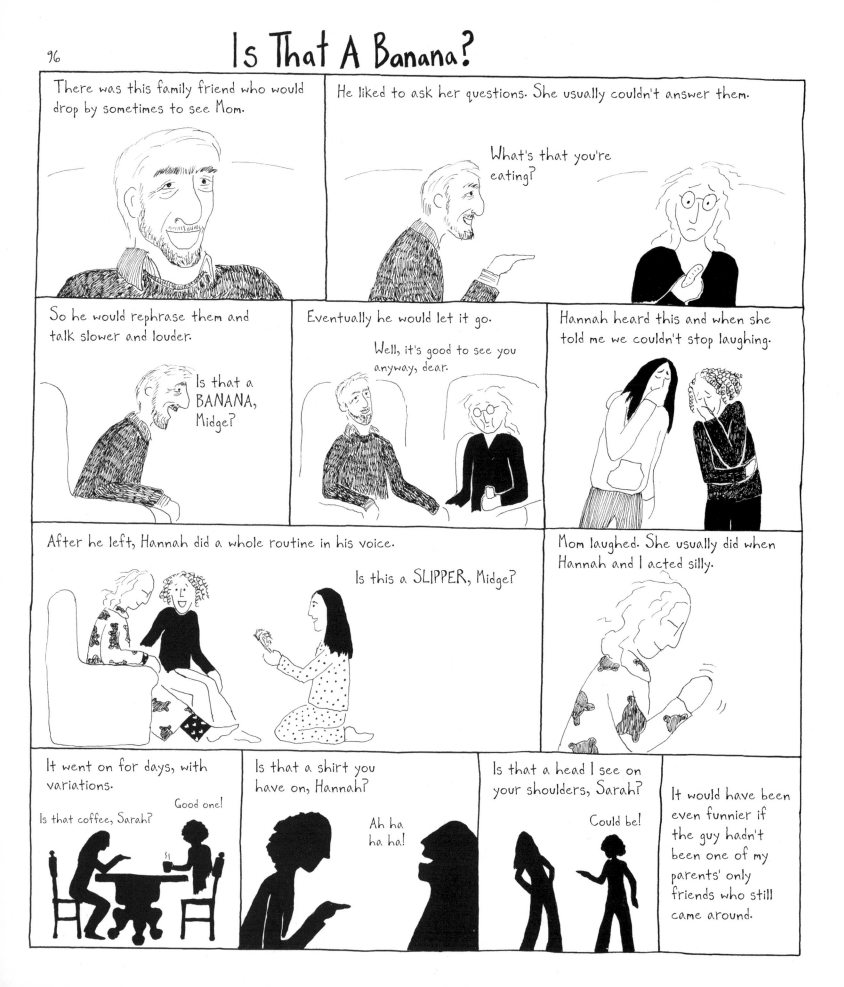

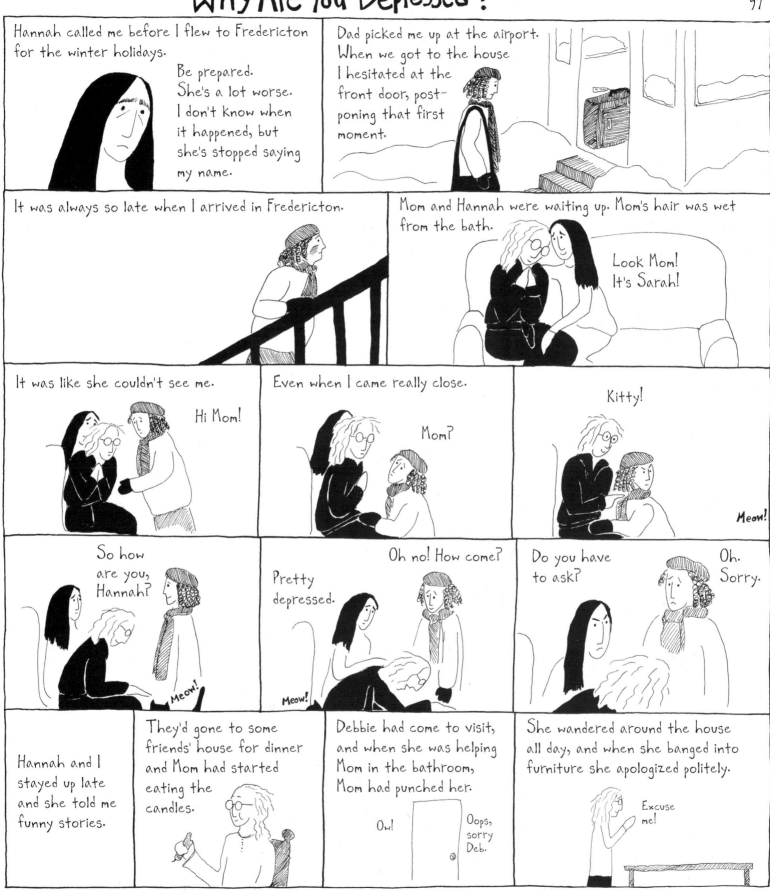

98

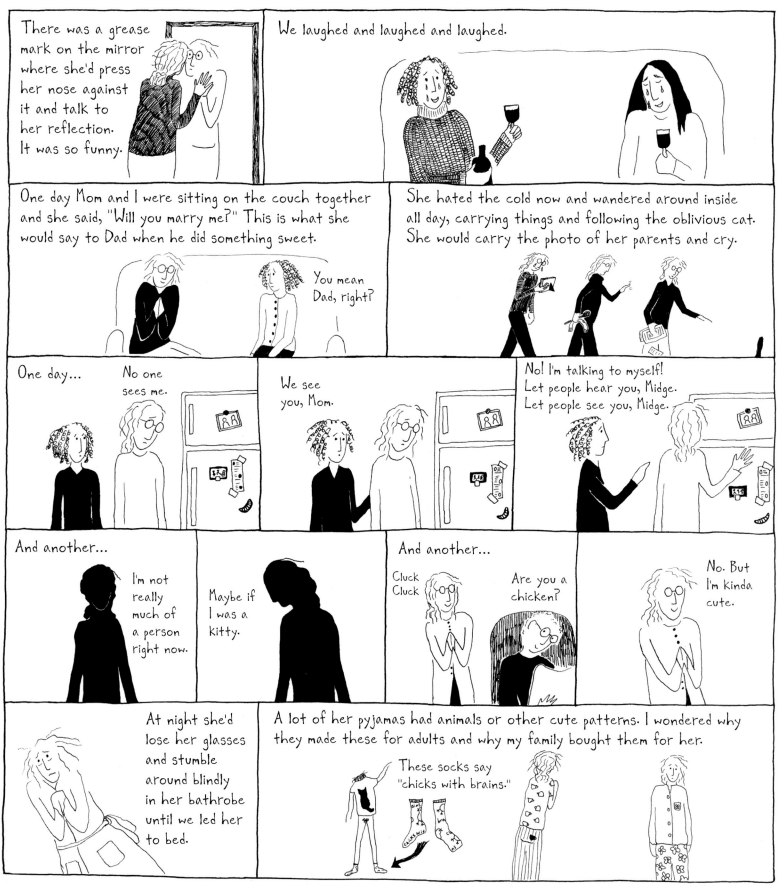

There was a grease mark on the mirror where she'd press her nose against it and talk to her reflection. It was so funny.

We laughed and laughed and laughed.

One day Mom and I were sitting on the couch together and she said, "Will you marry me?" This is what she would say to Dad when he did something sweet.

You mean Dad, right?

She hated the cold now and wandered around inside all day, carrying things and following the oblivious cat. She would carry the photo of her parents and cry.

One day... No one sees me.

We see you, Mom.

No! I'm talking to myself! Let people hear you, Midge. Let people see you, Midge.

And another... I'm not really much of a person right now.

Maybe if I was a kitty.

And another... Cluck Cluck

Are you a chicken?

No. But I'm kinda cute.

At night she'd lose her glasses and stumble around blindly in her bathrobe until we led her to bed.

A lot of her pyjamas had animals or other cute patterns. I wondered why they made these for adults and why my family bought them for her.

These socks say "chicks with brains."

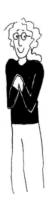

Who Farted?

Mom, Dad, and I were in the kitchen.
Hannah came in and said, "Ew! Who farted?"
Dad and I both denied it, and accused Hannah of
doing it herself. This went on for a while, until
Mom said in this sweet little voice, "No, I think I did."

We laughed so hard then, all four of us.

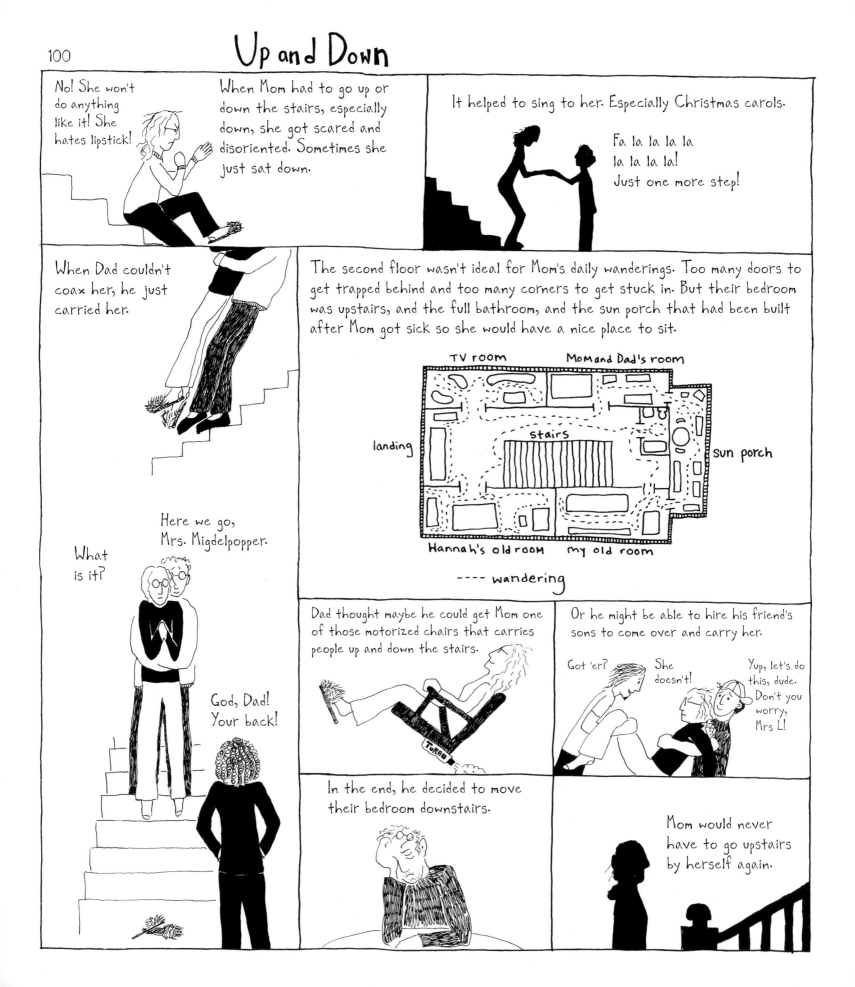

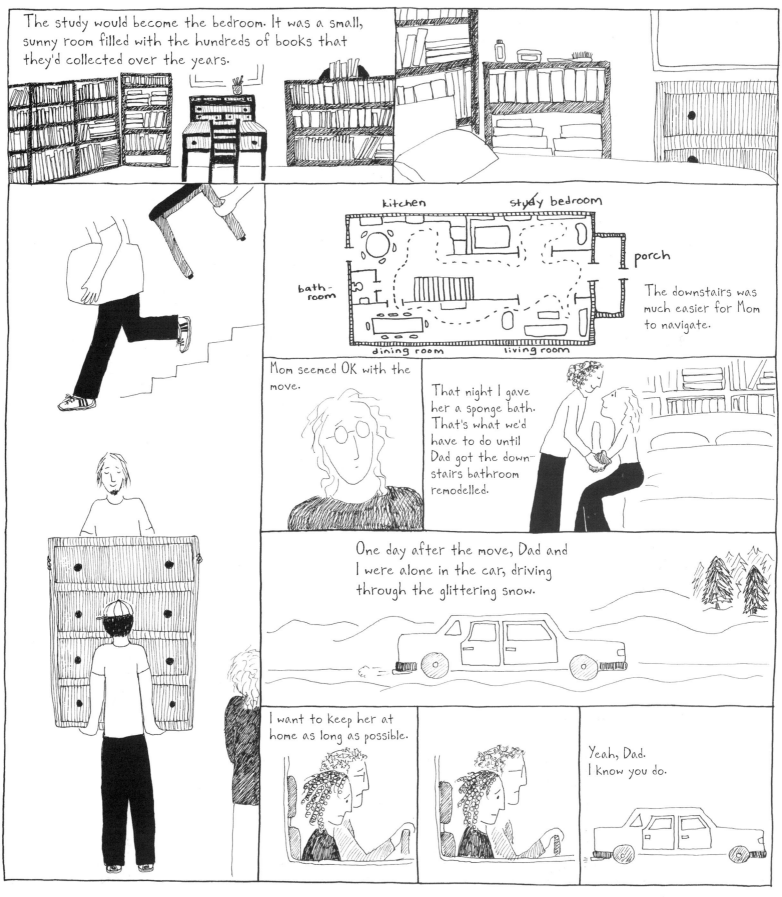

The study would become the bedroom. It was a small, sunny room filled with the hundreds of books that they'd collected over the years.

kitchen

study bedroom

porch

bath-room

The downstairs was much easier for Mom to navigate.

dining room

living room

Mom seemed OK with the move.

That night I gave her a sponge bath. That's what we'd have to do until Dad got the down-stairs bathroom remodelled.

One day after the move, Dad and I were alone in the car, driving through the glittering snow.

I want to keep her at home as long as possible.

Yeah, Dad. I know you do.

We still helped Mom go up and down the stairs sometimes, for a bath or a visit to the sun porch. The rest of the time we kept a baby gate at the bottom of the stairs just in case. But she mostly ignored them.

One day I was sitting at the top of the steps looking down at Mom and Dad.

She doesn't even know who I am, Dad.

Yes, she does. You know who Sarah is, right?

She never answered.

At some point, I don't know when or how or why, Dad had become extremely patient with Mom.

He held her hand and called her little nicknames.

Mom would say "I love you" over and over and he always said it back.

Sometimes they were so deep in their own little tender world that I had to leave them.

One day Mom and I were in the sun porch listening to Aretha Franklin.

Mmm Mmm Mmm

♪ Chain Chain ~ Chain Chain of Fools! ♪

Mom introduced me to her music when I was a kid and we both loved it.

I was thinking about how good the sun porch was for Mom.

Then she turned to me and said, "Who are you?"

Your daughter, Sarah.

My answer seemed to stress her out. She turned away and started mumbling and breathing heavily. That was the only time she ever said anything like that. Part of me wondered if she was joking or something.

Phew!

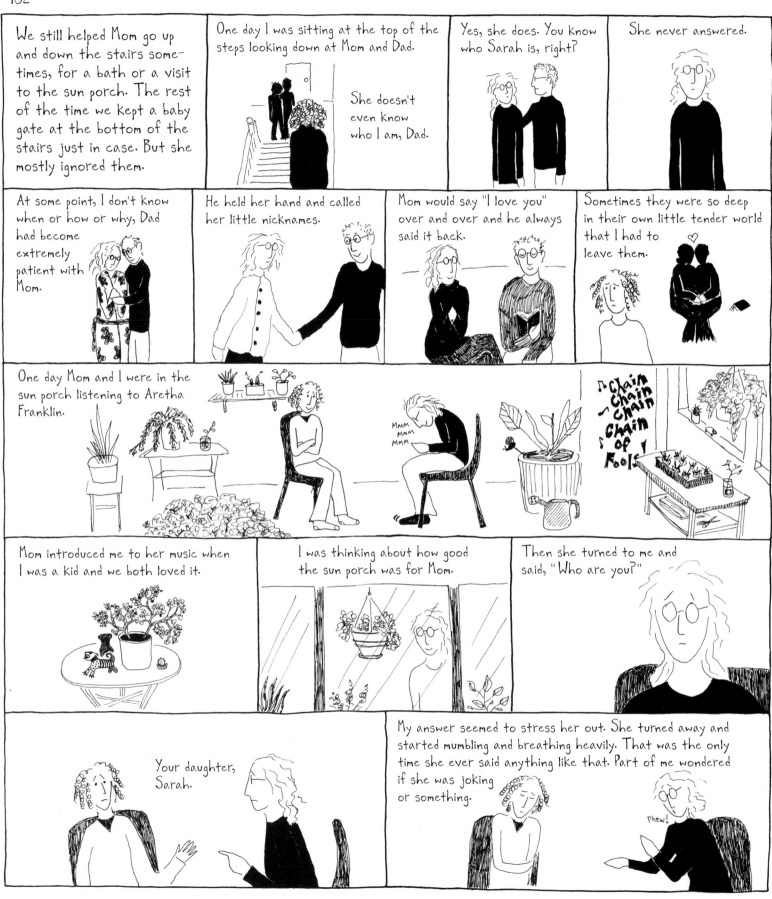

Oh Broccoli, Who Are Simple

Mom, Dad, and I were all sitting at the table. As usual,
Dad and I were trying to get Mom to eat more.

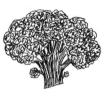

Sarah: Here Mom, it's broccoli from someone's garden!
Mom: Oh broccoli, who are simple!
Sarah: It would make me so happy if you ate this little
bit of food, Mom.
Dad: It's a morsellette. Can a morsel be anything besides food?
Sarah: I don't know. Maybe poetry.

[Pause]

Sarah: So is it only broccoli and carrot sticks now?
Dad: And candy. Midge, man cannot live on bread alone...
Oh, but I don't know about woman.
Sarah: Oh broccoli, who are simple.
Dad: What?
Sarah: Mom said that.
Dad: She did?
Sarah: Dad, you were sitting right here!
Mom: I love it! It's great, like blockers.
Dad: Midge, did you really apostrophize the broccoli?
Sarah: Oh look! Another person. I have one too.
She said that last night.
Dad: What did she say about broccoli again?
Sarah: Oh broccoli, who are simple.
Dad: Well, it is grammatically correct.

Popping Up

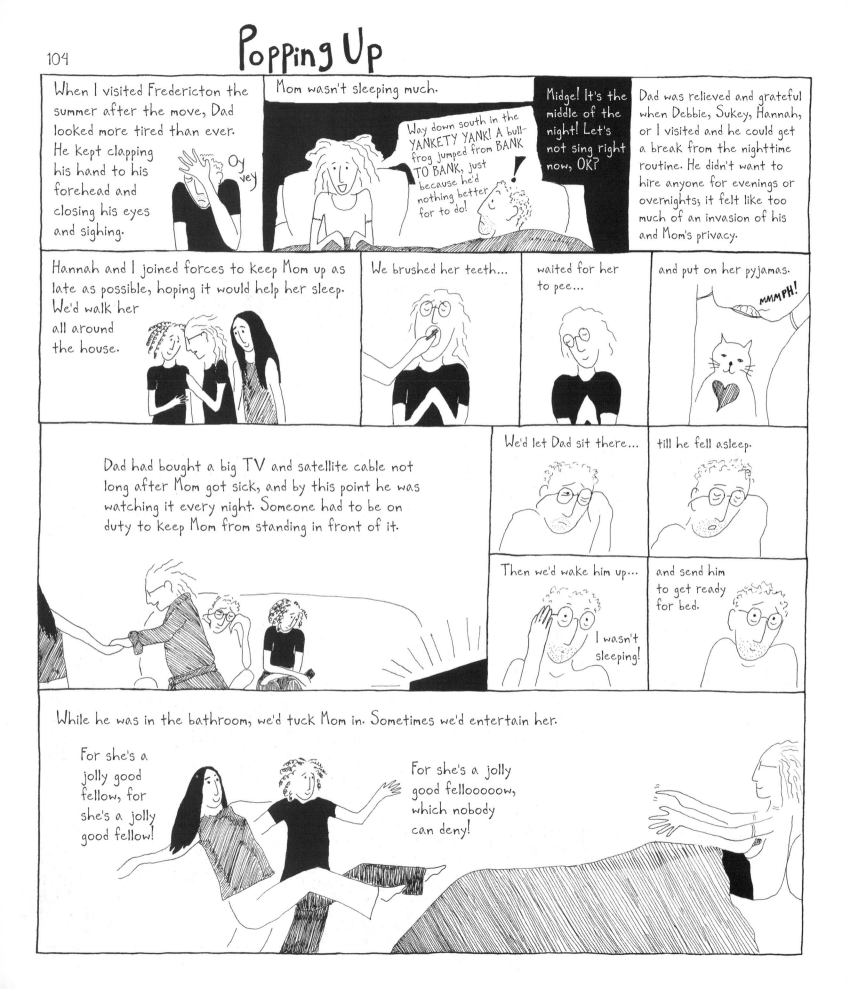

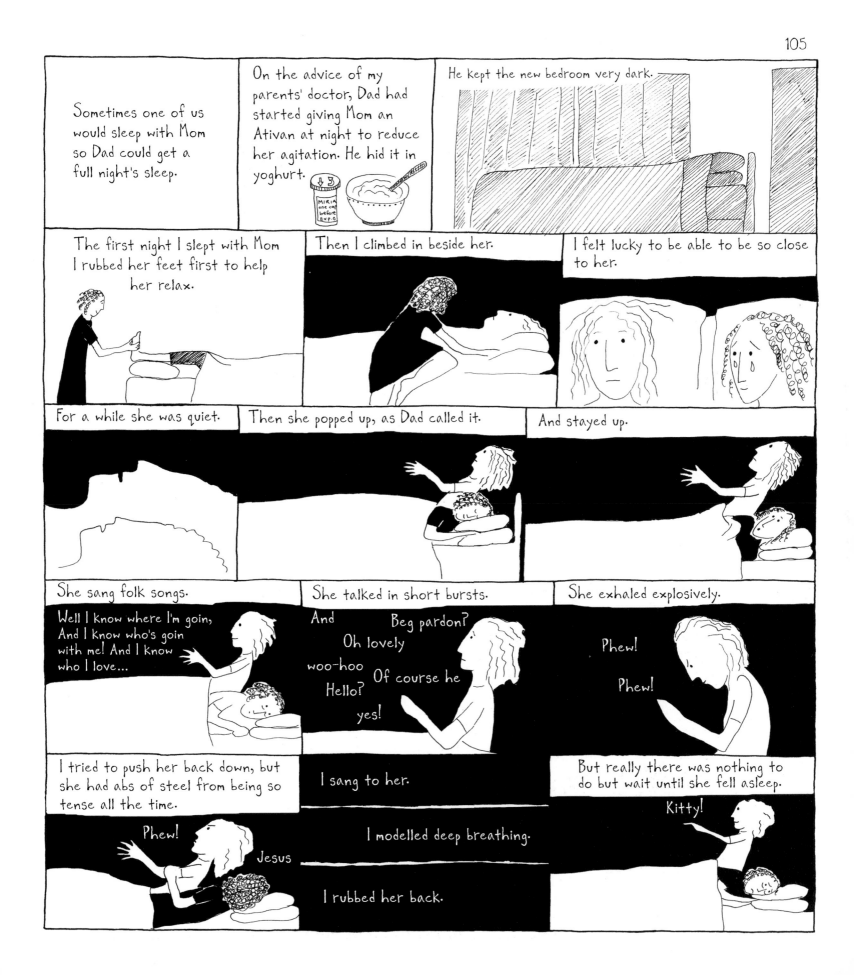

Sometimes one of us would sleep with Mom so Dad could get a full night's sleep.

On the advice of my parents' doctor, Dad had started giving Mom an Ativan at night to reduce her agitation. He hid it in yoghurt.

He kept the new bedroom very dark.

The first night I slept with Mom I rubbed her feet first to help her relax.

Then I climbed in beside her.

I felt lucky to be able to be so close to her.

For a while she was quiet.

Then she popped up, as Dad called it.

And stayed up.

She sang folk songs.

Well I know where I'm goin, And I know who's goin with me! And I know who I love...

She talked in short bursts.

And Beg pardon? Oh lovely woo-hoo Hello? Of course he yes!

She exhaled explosively.

Phew!

Phew!

I tried to push her back down, but she had abs of steel from being so tense all the time.

Phew!

Jesus

I sang to her.

I modelled deep breathing.

I rubbed her back.

But really there was nothing to do but wait until she fell asleep.

Kitty!

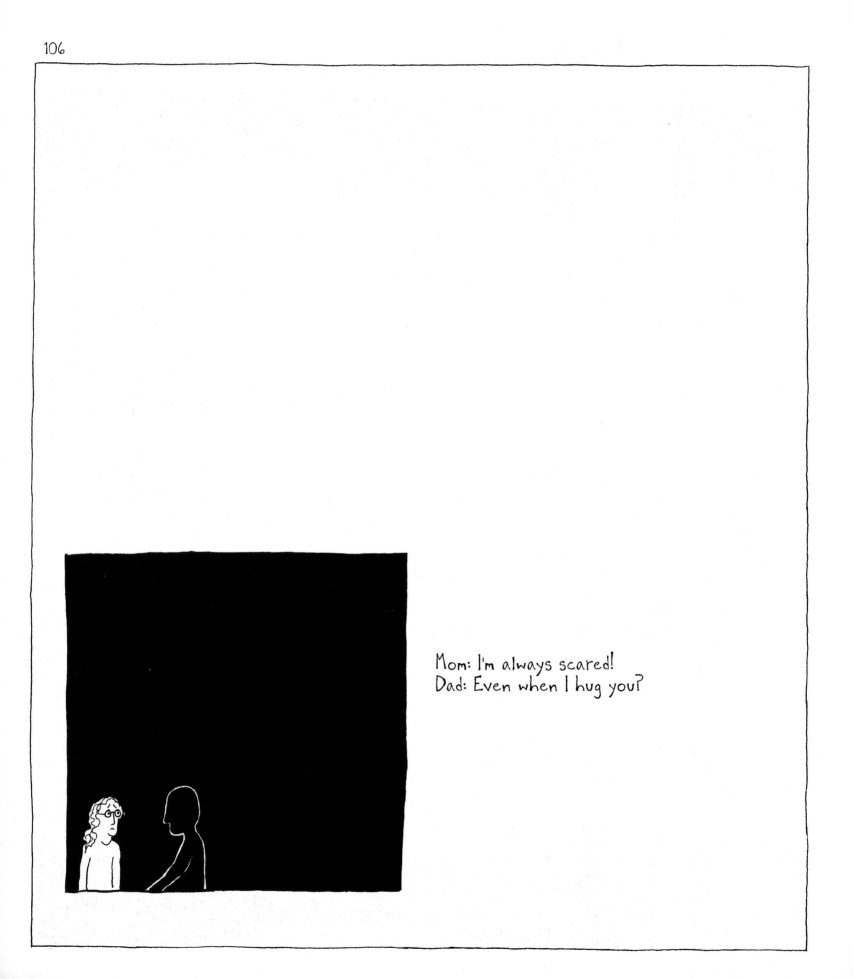

Mom: I'm always scared!
Dad: Even when I hug you?

Accidental

One night I was woken up by a huge crash.

I heard voices downstairs, but then I fell back asleep.

THUNK!

!

Ow!

Oh sweetie, let me help you up!

When I got up in the morning, Mom had a few scratches on her face. By the evening half her face was bruised and swollen. Dad called from work and told me she had fallen out of bed and smashed her face on the night table. I was furious. I'd told him a long time ago to get bed rails. I kept taking photos of her face. I couldn't believe it. She looked so bad. I couldn't tell if she noticed the injury. But she seemed sad.

Dad came home with some cheap plastic rails and I yelled at him.

Kidz SnapOn Rails
ONLY $19.99
KEEP YOUR CHILDREN SAFE
AGES 2-5, UP TO 50 lbs.

Stop making such a big deal out of it! These are fine for now. I'll order some better ones this week.

I left Fredericton a few days later.

The night before, I sat with Mom and held her. She seemed so fragile with her bruised face.

After she went to bed, Dad and I talked in the kitchen.

Thanks for everything.

I will.

It's OK, Dad. Just please get some rails, OK?

I left the house around four in the morning. Dad kept thanking me over and over.

As the taxi drove along the river to the airport, the snow got heavier until there was almost no visibility. The driver told me how much he loved driving and how he would stop sometimes to take pictures of beautiful snow formations or rainbows or sunrises. He also took pictures of car accidents and sent them to the paper. He got $40 for every one they printed.

TAXI

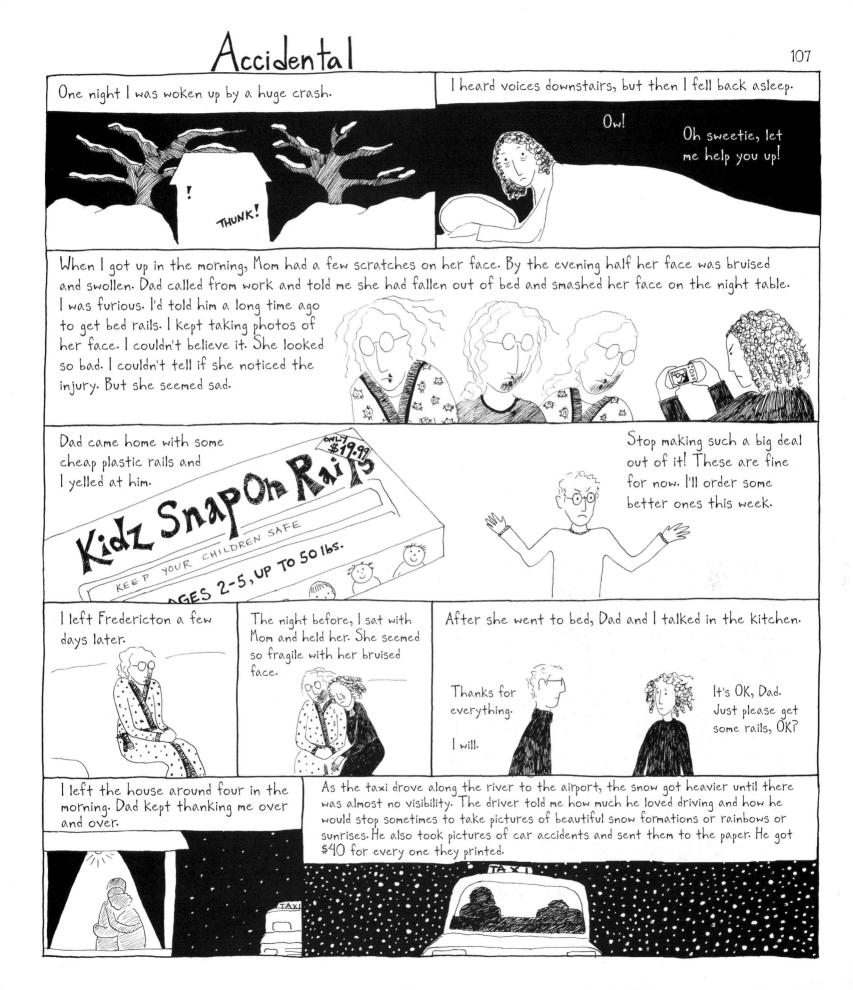

Lighter

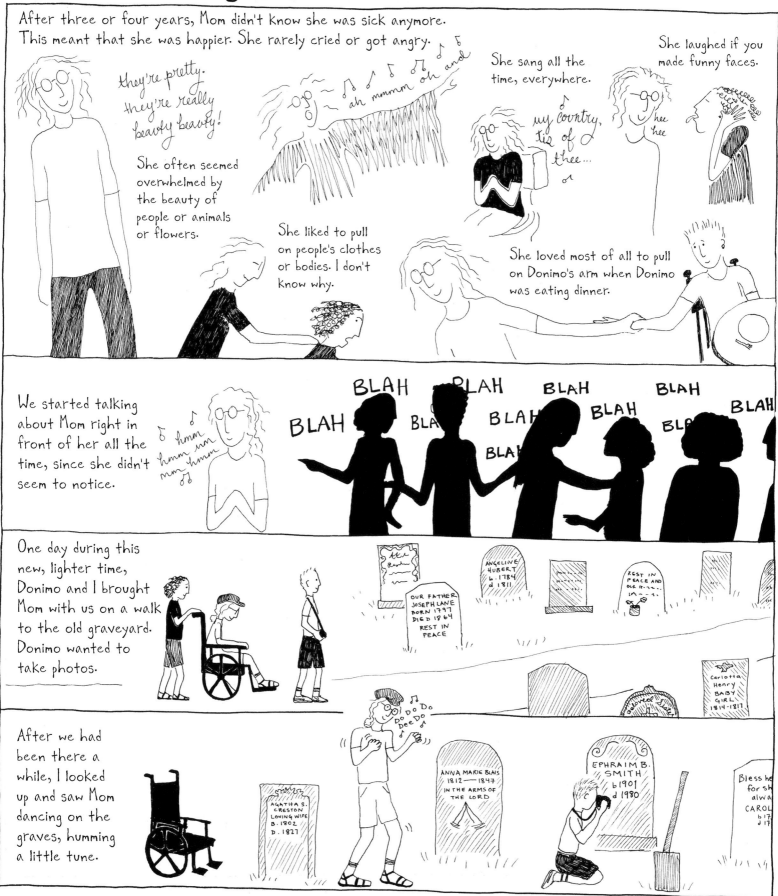

After three or four years, Mom didn't know she was sick anymore. This meant that she was happier. She rarely cried or got angry.

they're pretty. they're really beauty beauty!

She often seemed overwhelmed by the beauty of people or animals or flowers.

ah mmmm oh and

She sang all the time, everywhere.

my country, tis of thee...

thee hee

She laughed if you made funny faces.

She liked to pull on people's clothes or bodies. I don't know why.

She loved most of all to pull on Donimo's arm when Donimo was eating dinner.

We started talking about Mom right in front of her all the time, since she didn't seem to notice.

hmm um hmm um um hmm

BLAH BLAH BLAH BLAH BLAH BLAH BLAH BLAH BLAH

One day during this new, lighter time, Donimo and I brought Mom with us on a walk to the old graveyard. Donimo wanted to take photos.

OUR FATHER JOSEPH LANE BORN 1797 DIED 1864 REST IN PEACE

ANGELINE HUBERT b. 1784 d. 1811

REST IN PEACE AND OUR

Carlotta Henry BABY GIRL 1814-1817

After we had been there a while, I looked up and saw Mom dancing on the graves, humming a little tune.

Do Do Do Do Dee Do

AGATHA S. CRESTON LOVING WIFE B. 1802 D. 1827

ANNA MARIE BLAIS 1812 — 1847 IN THE ARMS OF THE LORD

EPHRAIM B. SMITH b 1901 d 1980

Bless he for sh alwa CAROL b 17 d 17

Dad would sing to Mom to get her to take her pills or eat.

"Swallow the yellow brick pill!

Swallow the yellow brick pill!"

Good Grooming

By the time Mom started wearing diapers, she was too out of it to notice or care.

We tried to make sure they didn't stick up out of her pants.

We still took her to the bathroom regularly. The diapers were for overnight and backup during the day. She often sang while she sat.

She was so docile. She submitted to tooth brushing, nose wiping, hair brushing.

She sat on the bench in the new bathroom while we bathed her. We gave her a washcloth to hold.

Often the diaper leaked overnight and we would have to strip all the sheets and the mattress pad. We did laundry almost every day.

There were supplies everywhere.

soft 'n' fresh

Sometimes I felt like the calmest, most capable nurse.

SARAH

Other times I thought I might throw up from the smell of urine or shit.

Hannah and I decided that it would be easier to keep Mom clean if we trimmed her pubic hair. It was very long. I held Mom in place while Hannah knelt in front of her with the scissors.

hmm hmm hmm

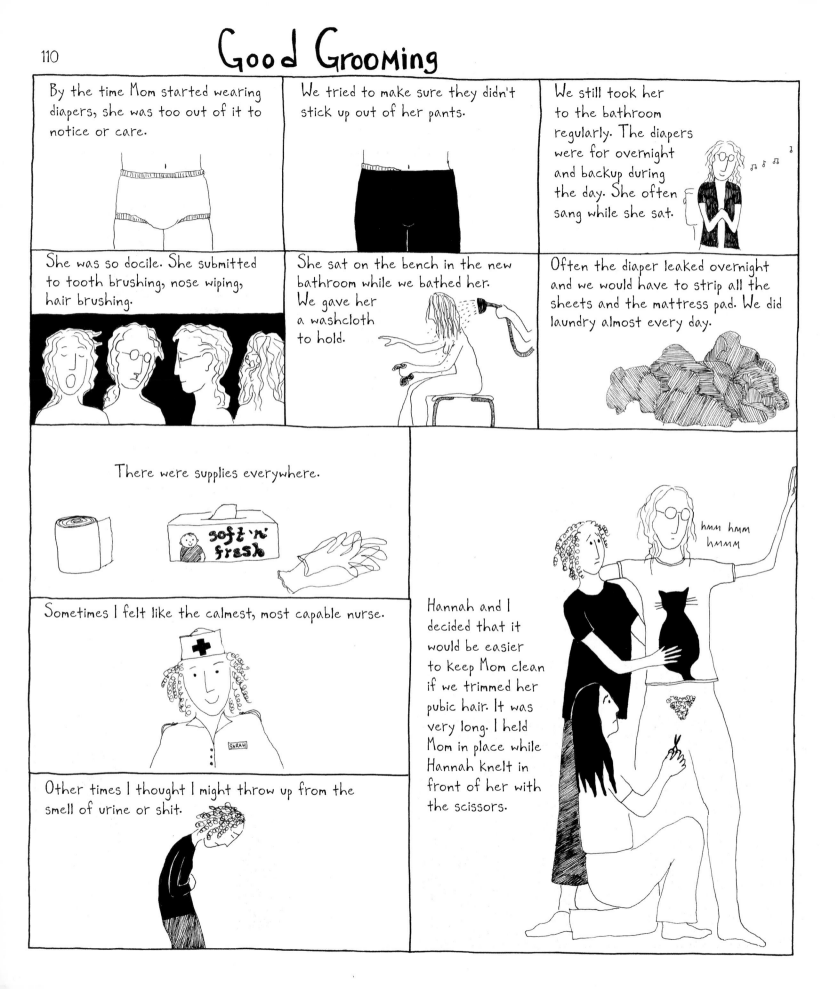

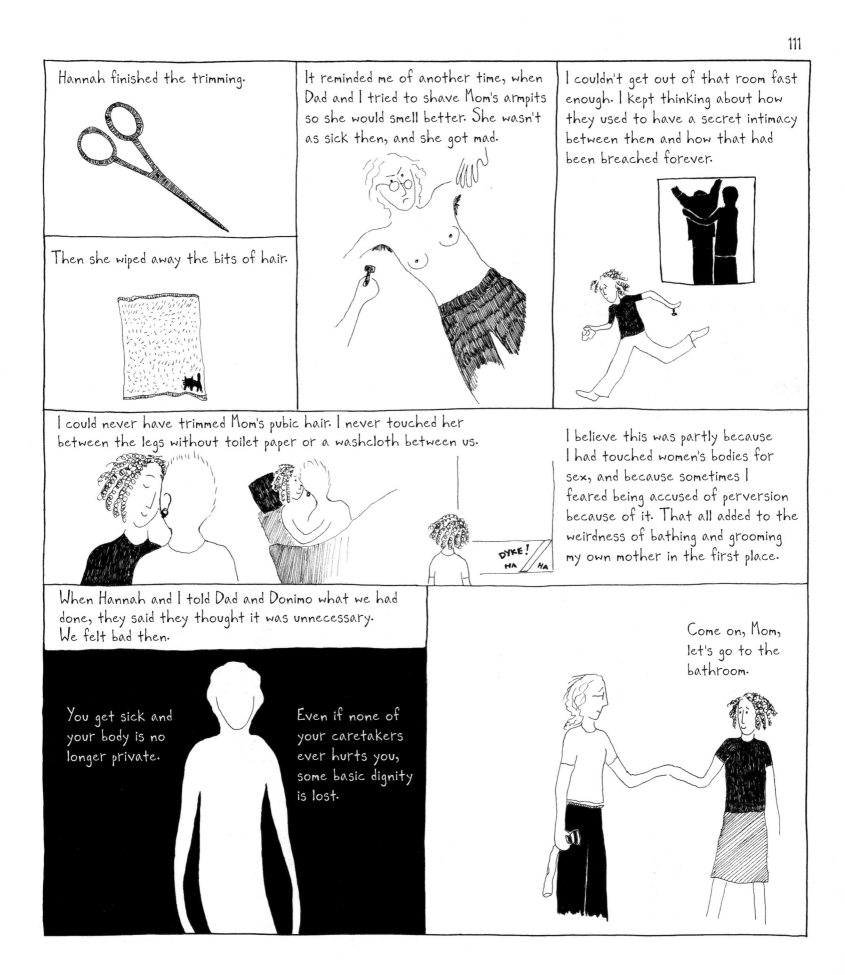

Hannah finished the trimming.

Then she wiped away the bits of hair.

It reminded me of another time, when Dad and I tried to shave Mom's armpits so she would smell better. She wasn't as sick then, and she got mad.

I couldn't get out of that room fast enough. I kept thinking about how they used to have a secret intimacy between them and how that had been breached forever.

I could never have trimmed Mom's pubic hair. I never touched her between the legs without toilet paper or a washcloth between us.

DYKE!
HA HA

I believe this was partly because I had touched women's bodies for sex, and because sometimes I feared being accused of perversion because of it. That all added to the weirdness of bathing and grooming my own mother in the first place.

When Hannah and I told Dad and Donimo what we had done, they said they thought it was unnecessary. We felt bad then.

You get sick and your body is no longer private.

Even if none of your caretakers ever hurts you, some basic dignity is lost.

Come on, Mom, let's go to the bathroom.

The Great Social Experiment

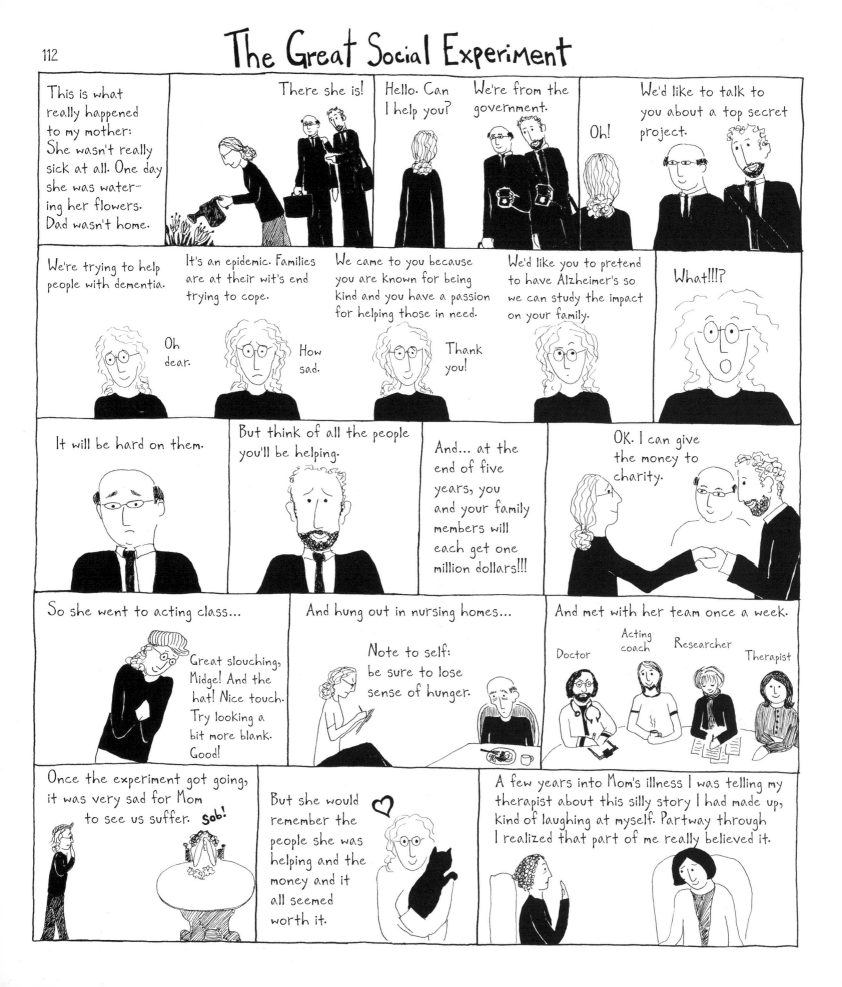

Scraps

Sarah: Oh my God!
Mom: (to the tune of Clementine)
Oh my Goddin, oh my Goddin...
Sarah: (laughs)
Mom: Don't. They can't help it if they
don't have enough.

Mom: I say that's little and she can but meanwhile.

Mom: (looking in mirror) This is live.
But it's OK, don't you think?

Sarah: Mom, did you eat the rye cracker?
Mom: No, it's eejier and squiggy to them.

Mom: Something's gonna happen to it.
Nice or not nice, nicely or lovely.

New

In the spring of 2004, Hannah had a baby and named him Zev.

Dad was overjoyed. As for Mom, it seemed like sometimes she caught a glimpse of him, and she'd smile. But mostly she didn't respond to him at all.

I talked to Hannah on the phone when she was up in the middle of the night with Zev.

I miss Mom so much! She would have been happier than anyone else to have a new baby in the family!

In the summer, Donimo and I went to visit.

Oh, how I craved my mother! I looked at her and touched her all the time, trying to soak her into my brain, my heart, my skin.

I rubbed her dry feet with cream.

I tried to untangle her hair.

She didn't touch me back, but she smiled.

Donimo and I didn't really understand the fuss about babies. We preferred our animals.

But we did fall in love with Zev.

We played a game where we flapped his big ears and pretended he could fly.

Mom woke up soaked in urine, in spite of the diaper. Sometimes even her shirt was wet. During the night she would wedge her arm or leg between the mattress and the bed rails and lie there trapped.

She didn't speak much. Her glasses fell off or she pulled them off. Her dark eyes darted like a scared animal's.

Donimo stayed alone with Mom for the first time.

Have a carrot!

Oh Christ!

"Your mom's mind is like the garden this summer," Donimo said.

"Tangled, but with spots of brightness."

Sometimes I craved my mother. Other times I fled her illness and escaped to Zev's new life.

Hello, cute thing!

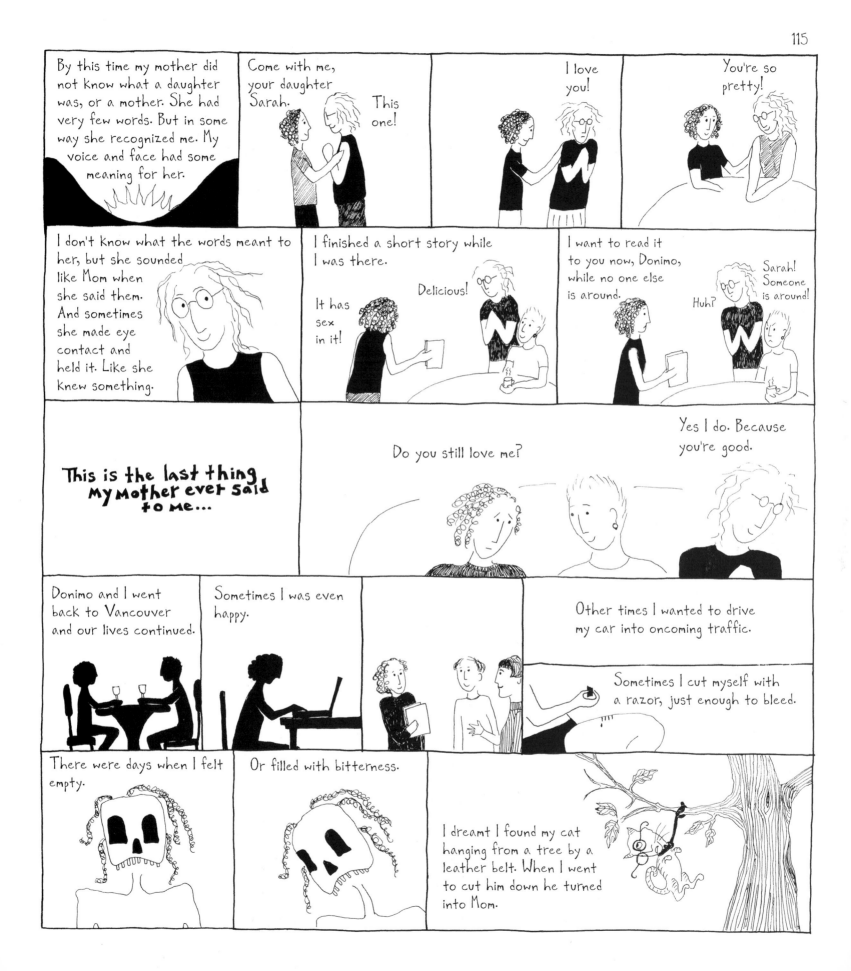

Decision

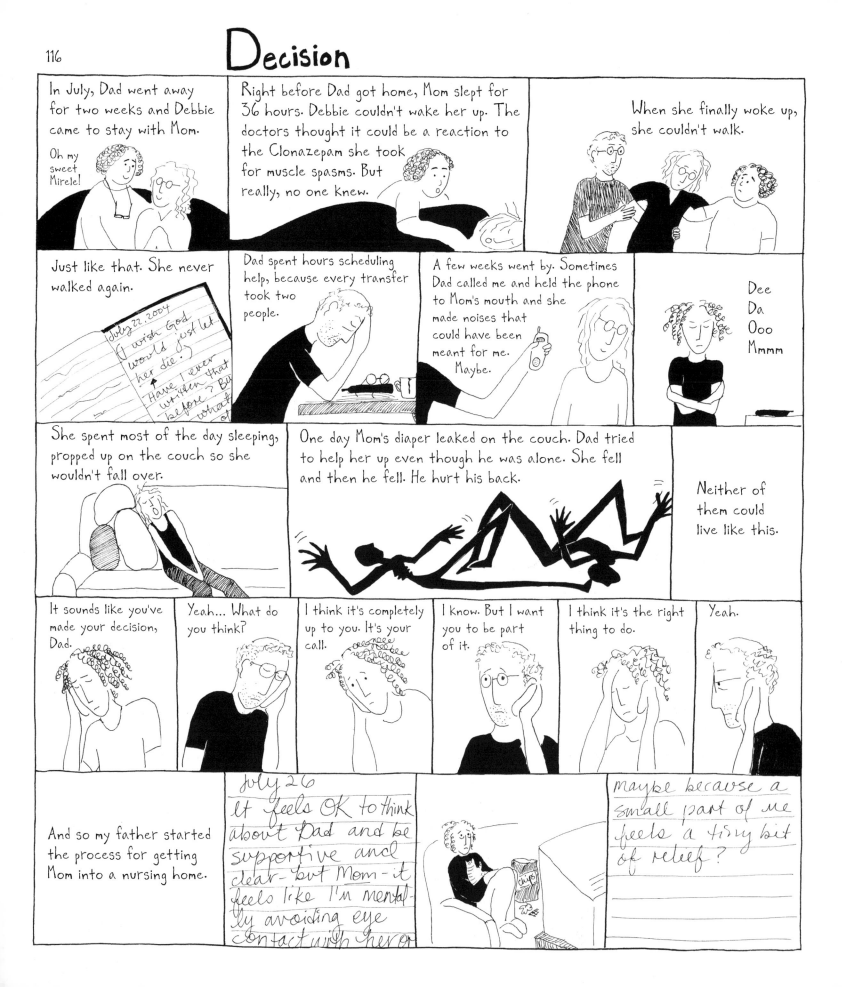

In July, Dad went away for two weeks and Debbie came to stay with Mom.

Oh my sweet Mirele!

Right before Dad got home, Mom slept for 36 hours. Debbie couldn't wake her up. The doctors thought it could be a reaction to the Clonazepam she took for muscle spasms. But really, no one knew.

When she finally woke up, she couldn't walk.

Just like that. She never walked again.

July 22, 2004
(I wish God would just let her die.)
Have I ever written that before? But what of

Dad spent hours scheduling help, because every transfer took two people.

A few weeks went by. Sometimes Dad called me and held the phone to Mom's mouth and she made noises that could have been meant for me. Maybe.

Dee
Da
Ooo
Mmmm

She spent most of the day sleeping, propped up on the couch so she wouldn't fall over.

One day Mom's diaper leaked on the couch. Dad tried to help her up even though he was alone. She fell and then he fell. He hurt his back.

Neither of them could live like this.

It sounds like you've made your decision, Dad.

Yeah... What do you think?

I think it's completely up to you. It's your call.

I know. But I want you to be part of it.

I think it's the right thing to do.

Yeah.

And so my father started the process for getting Mom into a nursing home.

July 26
It feels OK to think about Dad and be supportive and clear- but Mom - it feels like I'm mentally avoiding eye contact with her or

maybe because a small part of me feels a tiny bit of relief?

I spent a lot of time doing nothing, lying in bed with my cat Oscar.

Or trying to pick fights with Donimo.

I had trouble doing the most basic tasks. I often wondered if I had Alzheimer's too.

I kept going to work because it seemed like that's what people did, even when the world was falling apart.

In August Dad got a call. There was an opening for Mom in a nursing home. It was the one Dad had hoped to get her into: small, with excellent staff. But she had to move in in two days.

Dad said he was ready. He described how he was going to rearrange the furniture after Mom was gone. He seemed desperate for freedom.

AAAAAHHHH!

Hannah wrote that she hoped Dad could wrap this up fast so that she and Dad and Zev could go on the trip they'd planned.

On a trip to Vancouver the year before, Dad had bought a glass egg-shaped sculpture. He had always had to keep it hidden in case Mom broke it. When she stopped walking he put it out on display.

I would get really angry at Hannah and Dad and then wonder if I had any right, since I wasn't there doing the day-to-day.

Sukey came and she and Dad packed up Mom's things.

Wow. I guess she doesn't need much.

No.

Hannah came and brought Zev.

Look, Mom! It's your grandson!

On August 11, six days before her sixtieth birthday, Mom moved into Pine Grove.

Welcome!

Look at all the people today.

I went to work that day.

I kept calling them to see what was happening. They stayed with Mom all day, then went and got dinner, then came back for a while. Then they left.

Donimo and I made a little altar for Mom, with photos and rocks and shells and flowers.

We lit candles and said out loud what we wished for her in this new stage. Mostly we wanted her not to be scared.

Subsiding

Dad visited Mom almost every day.

Well hello again, dear!

Hi Sylvia. Nice to see you.

He'd find her in the common area; the nursing home made sure everyone got up and out of their rooms every day, unless they were sick.

Every day a worker would take the time to do Mom's hair in a neat ponytail or even braids.

She even got regular baths. They used some sort of hoist to get her in. She'd had only showers for so long.

She didn't really talk anymore. Dad brought poetry to read to her, books that had belonged to her in college and still had her notes in the margins.

They both loved e e cummings, even when he was "being fresh" as Mom used to call it.

the Cambridge ladies who live in furnished souls
are unbeautiful and have comfortable minds
(also, with the church's protestant blessings
daughters, unscented shapeless spirited)
they believe in Christ and Longfellow, both dead

They liked his romantic poems too...

when by now and tree by leaf
she laughed his joy she cried his grief
bird by snow and stir by still
anyone's any was all to her

And Robert Frost was Mom's favourite.

then leaf subsides to leaf

Every evening Dad would say good night to Mom and go home. He thought of bringing her with him to see the house and the kitty, but it didn't seem like she would notice. She seemed content where she was.

In the first little while, Mom would smile when Dad arrived.

Then more and more often she would be asleep.

After a month or so, he wasn't sure if she recognized him anymore.

Then one day, he told me, she looked right through him.

She ate less and less. She was less and less responsive.

After she'd been there only a couple months, she got an infection and was too weak to leave her bed.

She rallied for a bit, but then weakened again. No one could say for sure what was wrong.

They said she might not get better.

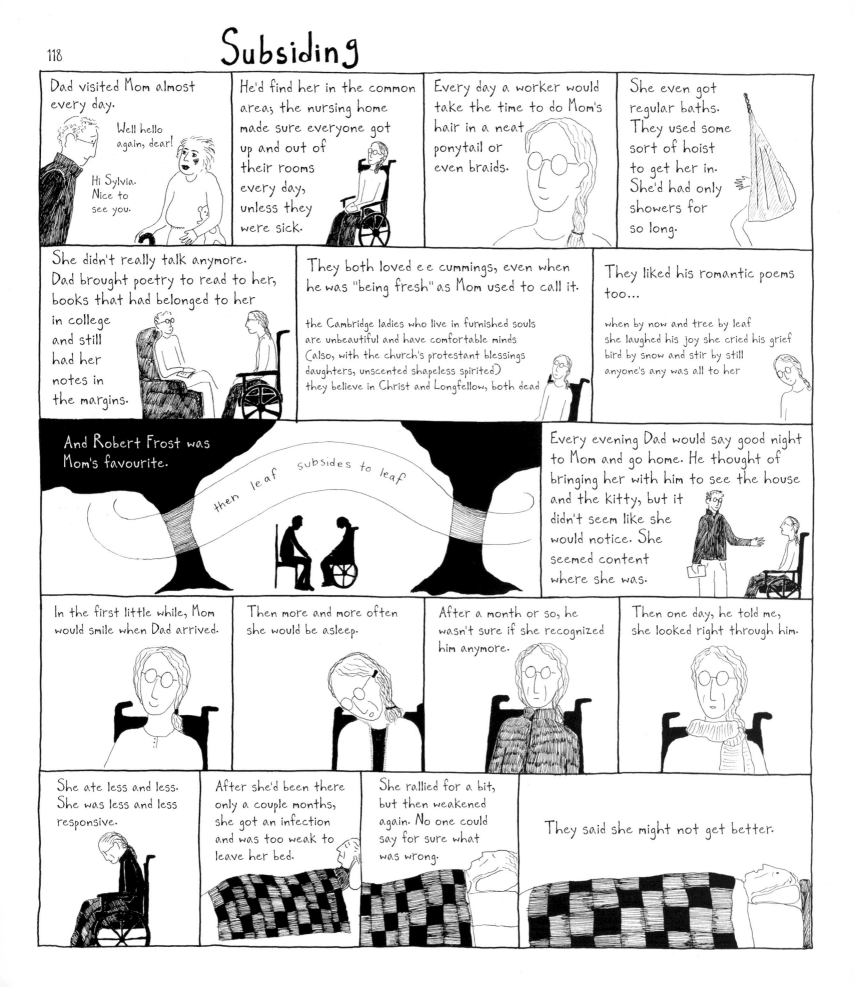

The End

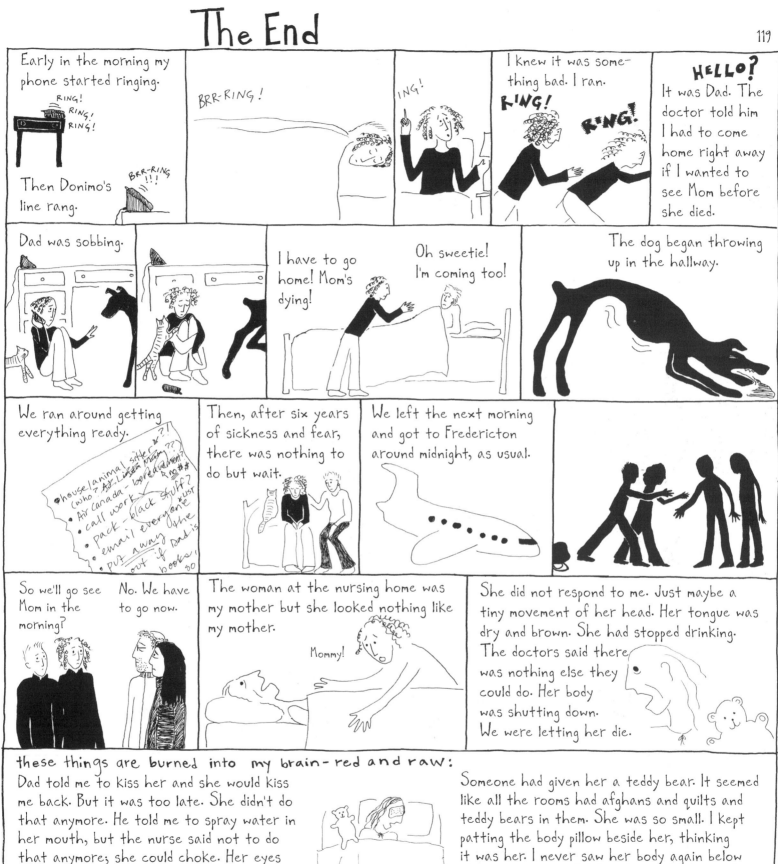

Early in the morning my phone started ringing.

RING! RING! RING!

Then Donimo's line rang.

BRR-RING!!!

BRR-RING!

ING!

I knew it was something bad. I ran.

RING!

RING!

HELLO? It was Dad. The doctor told him I had to come home right away if I wanted to see Mom before she died.

Dad was sobbing.

I have to go home! Mom's dying!

Oh sweetie! I'm coming too!

The dog began throwing up in the hallway.

We ran around getting everything ready.

Then, after six years of sickness and fear, there was nothing to do but wait.

We left the next morning and got to Fredericton around midnight, as usual.

So we'll go see Mom in the morning?

No. We have to go now.

The woman at the nursing home was my mother but she looked nothing like my mother.

Mommy!

She did not respond to me. Just maybe a tiny movement of her head. Her tongue was dry and brown. She had stopped drinking. The doctors said there was nothing else they could do. Her body was shutting down. We were letting her die.

these things are burned into my brain-red and raw:

Dad told me to kiss her and she would kiss me back. But it was too late. She didn't do that anymore. He told me to spray water in her mouth, but the nurse said not to do that anymore; she could choke. Her eyes would not close. We put a damp cloth on her forehead and sometimes over her eyes. Her mouth never closed either.

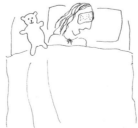

Someone had given her a teddy bear. It seemed like all the rooms had afghans and quilts and teddy bears in them. She was so small. I kept patting the body pillow beside her, thinking it was her. I never saw her body again below the neck, except for her hands. Dad said if I squeezed her hand, she would squeeze back. But it was too late for that, too.

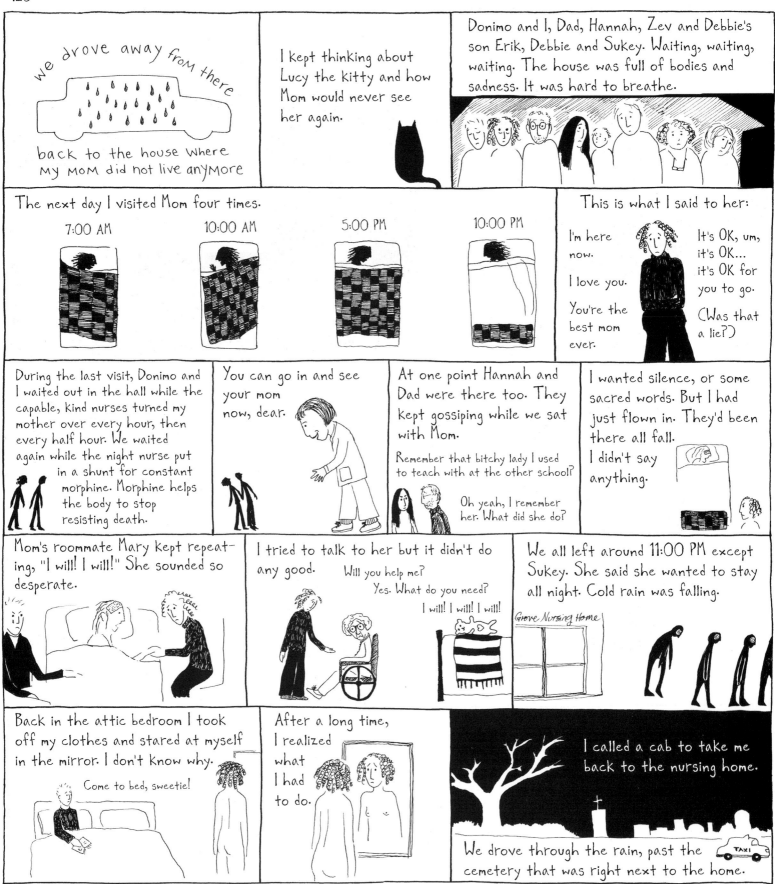

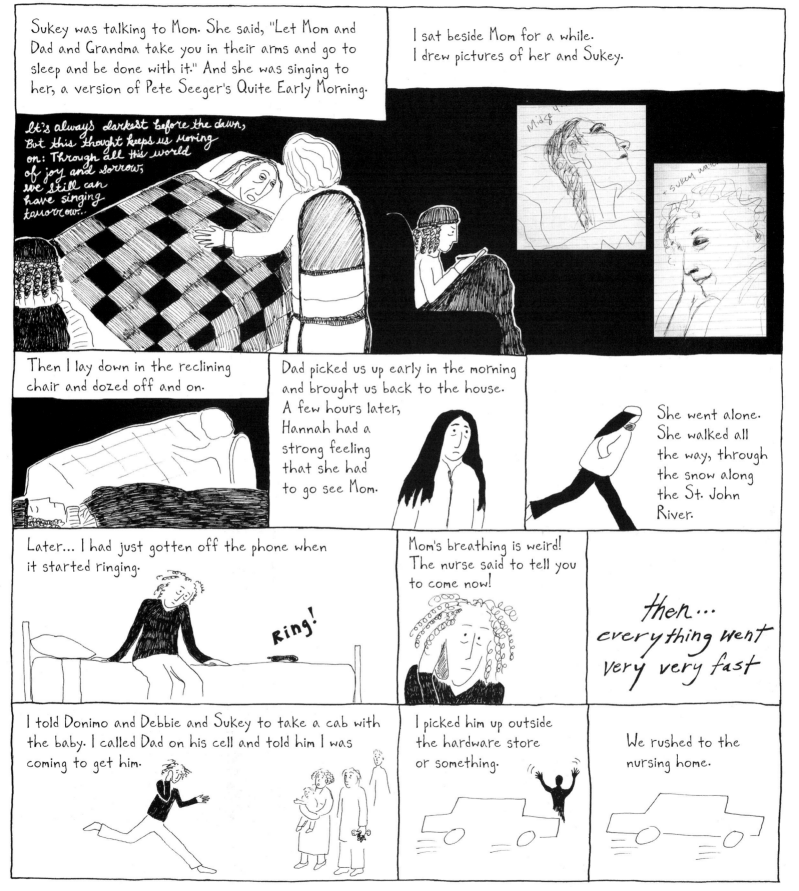

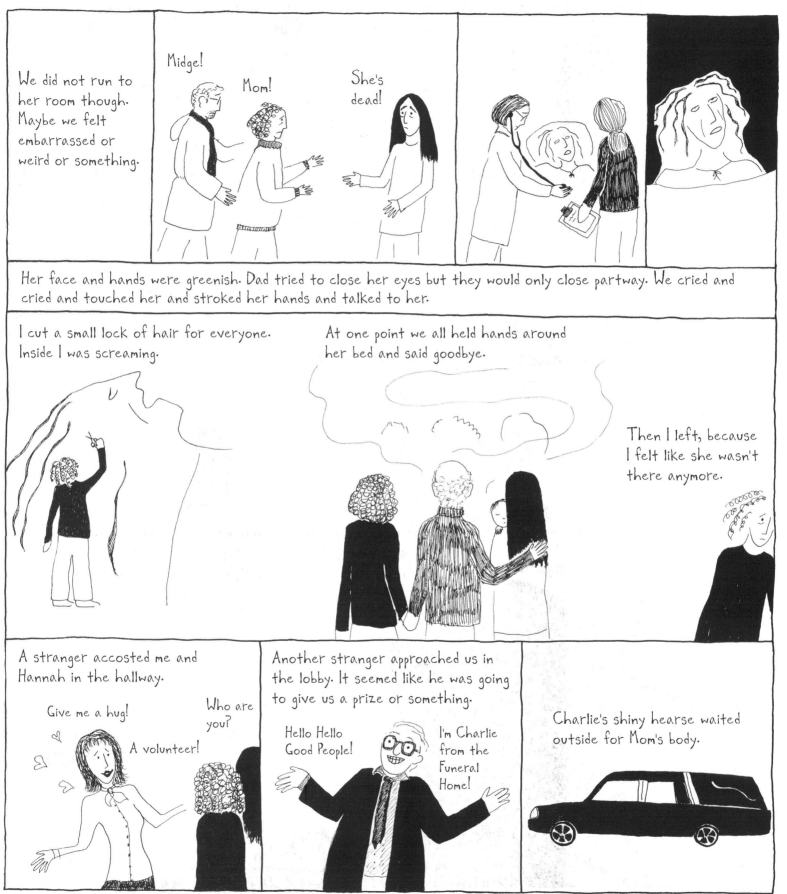

We did not run to her room though. Maybe we felt embarrassed or weird or something.

Midge!

Mom!

She's dead!

Her face and hands were greenish. Dad tried to close her eyes but they would only close partway. We cried and cried and touched her and stroked her hands and talked to her.

I cut a small lock of hair for everyone. Inside I was screaming.

At one point we all held hands around her bed and said goodbye.

Then I left, because I felt like she wasn't there anymore.

A stranger accosted me and Hannah in the hallway.

Give me a hug!

Who are you?

A volunteer!

Another stranger approached us in the lobby. It seemed like he was going to give us a prize or something.

Hello Hello Good People!

I'm Charlie from the Funeral Home!

Charlie's shiny hearse waited outside for Mom's body.

We all went back to Dad's house.

Shall not want.

He

We drank a lot of wine.

beside the still

waters.

I read aloud Psalm 23, which was Mom's favourite. Dad told us that. I didn't even know she read the Bible.

me in the paths of righteousness

Then I made two huge batches of chocolate chip cookies.

fear no evil:

There were no chips so I smashed up squares of Baker's chocolate.

comfort me.

We ate all the cookies.

runneth over.

Then I was so drunk I had to lie down under the kitchen table for a while.

Mercy

all the days of my life:

That night I wrapped myself in a shawl I had given Mom, dark blue cotton with a night sky print in white and turquoise.

Donimo and I lay in bed and I felt weird. I noticed the cat sitting on the dresser watching us.

She was so black and it was so dark that I couldn't see any of her features. She leapt down.

I propped myself up and got out my journal, like I had almost every night since my mother got sick.

there will be no more drawing, and I really thought there would be. Mom died today.

for ever.

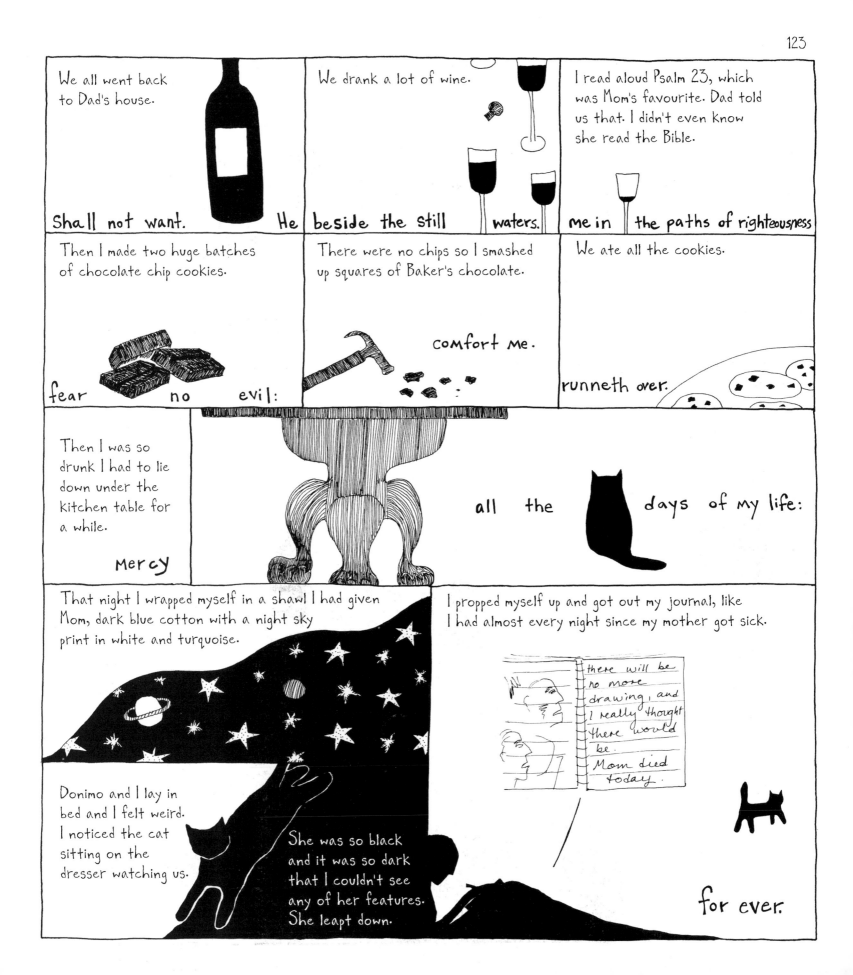

Next

That night or the next day, some old friends of Mom and Dad's showed up at the door. Dad invited them in for some wine.

Oh, Sarah, I'm so sorry about your mother!

It's too bad you didn't bother visiting while she was still alive!

Oh, we would have. It just always seemed like your Mom and Dad didn't want visitors.

Then I remembered that they had dropped by once. It was late at night. They put a casserole on the front steps, rang the doorbell, and drove away as fast as they could.

SCREECH!

I stomped upstairs. They stayed downstairs and drank Dad's wine unfazed.

That bitch! You told her!

Yeah.

The next day, we started planning the memorial. Debbie wanted more relatives to come and stay at Dad's house.

Ahem.

Debbie, I am sick of cooking and cleaning for everyone! We can't add even more people who don't lift a finger!

Fine. We'll just go back to New York and have our own memorial.

Oh for Christ's sake!

Later I apologized, because there was nothing else to do. We didn't publicize the memorial, because we didn't want people like the casserole droppers to come. In fact, very few of Mom and Dad's old friends ended up being invited.

Hannah made a poster and presented it like a teacher.

MIDGE

Dad read a Robert Frost poem and went through piles of Kleenex.

"once they are bowed/ So low for long, they never right themselves."

I can't remember what I said.

That night I apologized to Dad for yelling at people. "It's OK," he said. "It reminded me of Mom. You have this quality that she had. I always called it RADIANT BITCHINESS. It's a good quality to have."

Frost POEMS

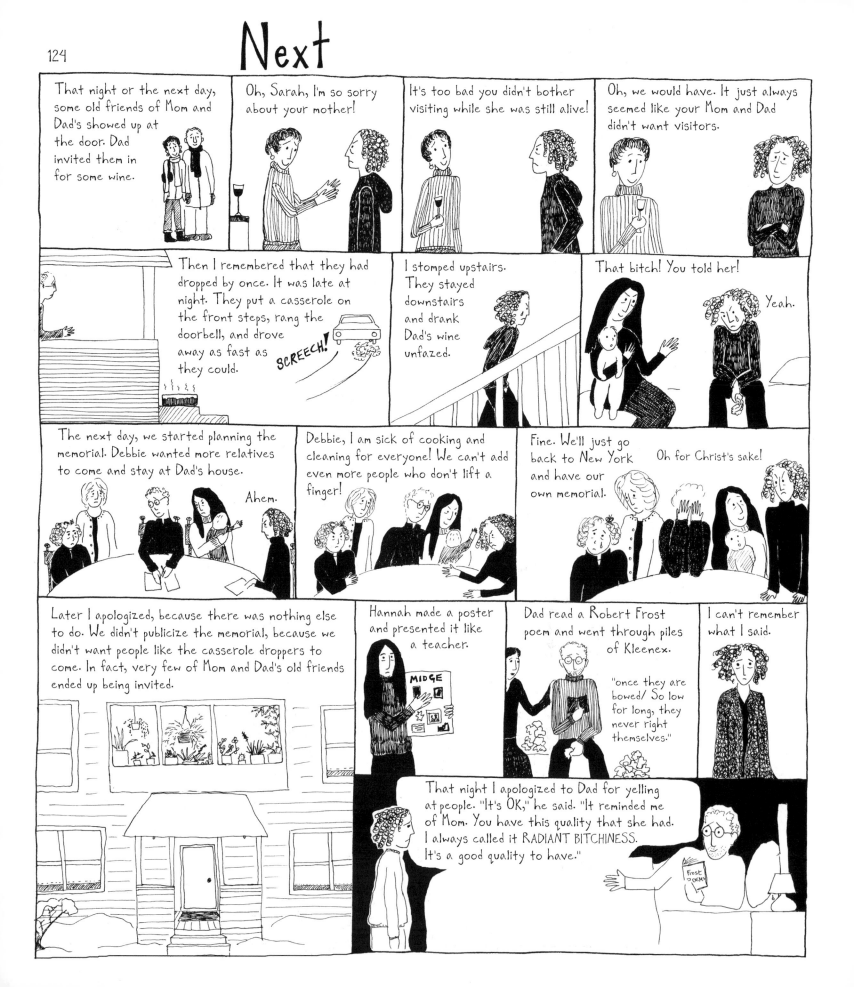

After

Mom did not believe in God.

I wasn't sure if I did or not, and when I did invoke his existence, I was usually angry at him. Sukey and I both reached our limit with him our last night with Mom.

In spite of this, I always knew I would say the mourner's Kaddish for Mom.

In Jewish tradition, you say Kaddish every day for 11 months after the death of a parent. The prayer itself is not about death or mourning. It affirms the mourner's faith in God. It shows that the mourner had good parents who instilled a strong faith that endures through great grief. I didn't care what the words were. I wanted the ritual.

I remembered the mourners who stood to say Kaddish in synagogue. I wanted to remember Mom every day like that.

The mourner says Kaddish surrounded by the congregation, who chime in at certain lines. The first few days of saying Kaddish, Donimo was my congregation. We sat on the floor of the attic and read the transliterated Hebrew together. I wrapped myself in the blanket I had given Mom.

The day after I first said Kaddish, I went running in Odell Park. They didn't keep deer there anymore. As I ran through the empty woods, I felt Mom in the trees. It was as if the air got denser and pressed against me. It only lasted a few seconds. I felt scared and grateful all at once.

Hannah carried Mom's ashes back from the funeral home. After she told me they were very heavy, I couldn't bring myself to hold them. Dad put them in a wooden box on his dresser. He put three amethysts on top for me and him and Hannah.

Donimo and I said Kaddish every night.

Many times a day I was knocked off my feet by the absolute absence of my mother.

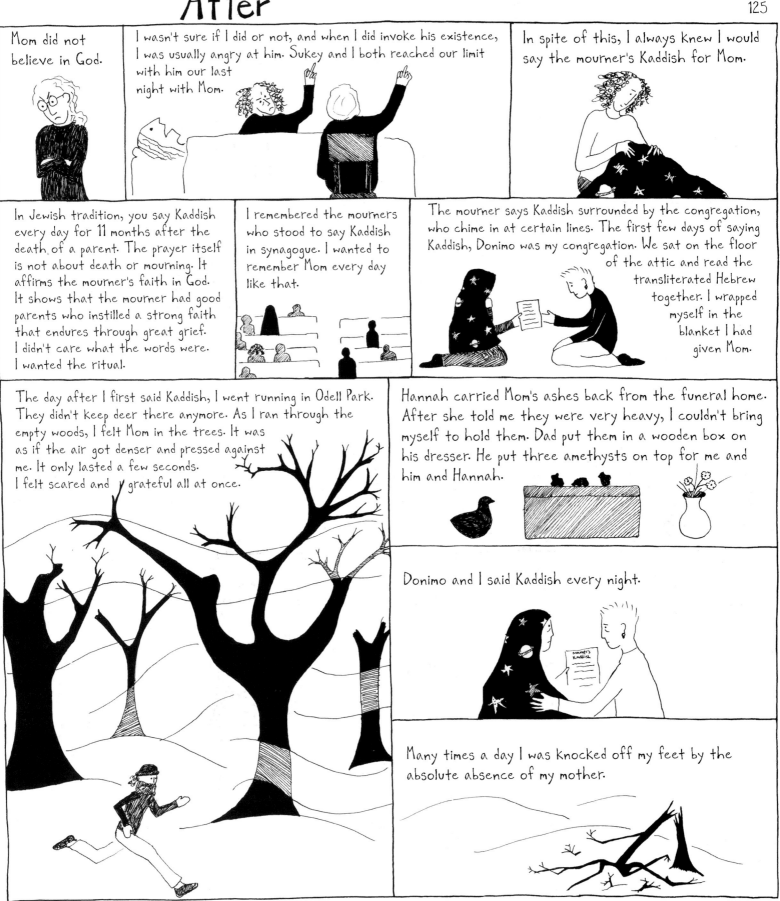

One day when I was alone in the house, I finally touched the box of ashes.

The air around it felt thick, like in Odell Park.

Dad and I took the toilet seat and the shower chair back to the rental place. We got rid of the bed rails too.

Donimo went home to Vancouver and I said Kaddish alone for the first time.

We packed up the things of Mom's that no one in the family wanted. "I can't believe it's all over," Dad said.

I kept thinking about all the time I spent trying to soak her up when she was alive. How every second had been important.

I said Kaddish. I covered my head and stretched myself out on the floor and cried. I made the Kaddish into my own prayer, my time I spent with her every night.

Every day I mourned the loss of her blazing, protective love.

The words of the Kaddish and the feeling of the cloth against my skin and the solidity of the floor against my forehead comforted me every night.

It helped to think about saying Kaddish for 11 months, and to realize that some day I would say the prayer for my mother for the last time. Each time I said the Kaddish was precious. And some day I wouldn't need to say it anymore.

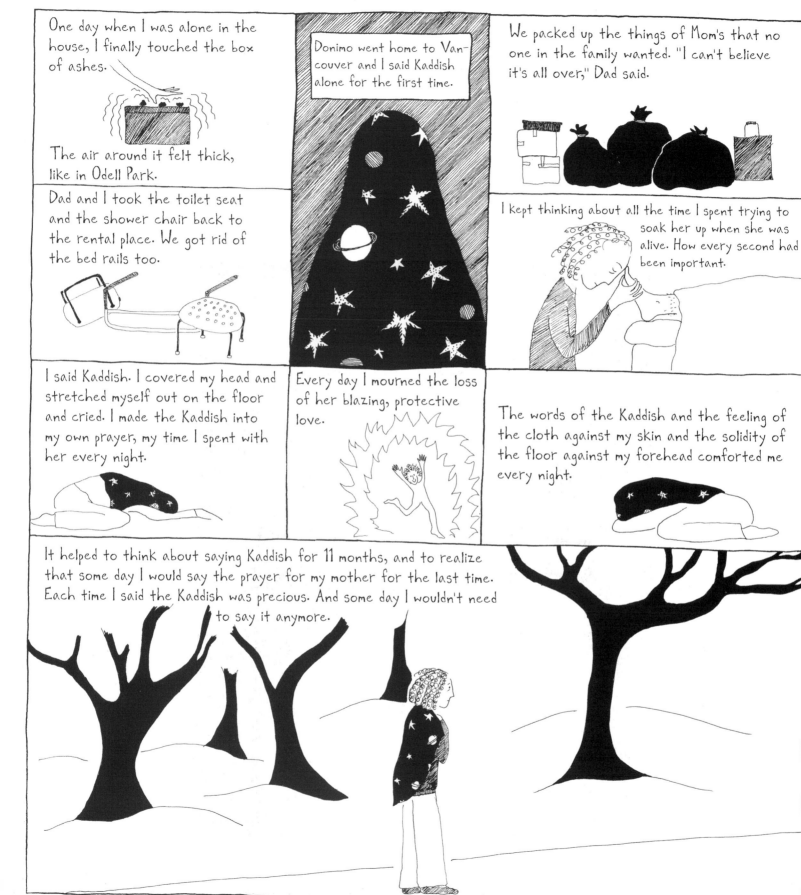

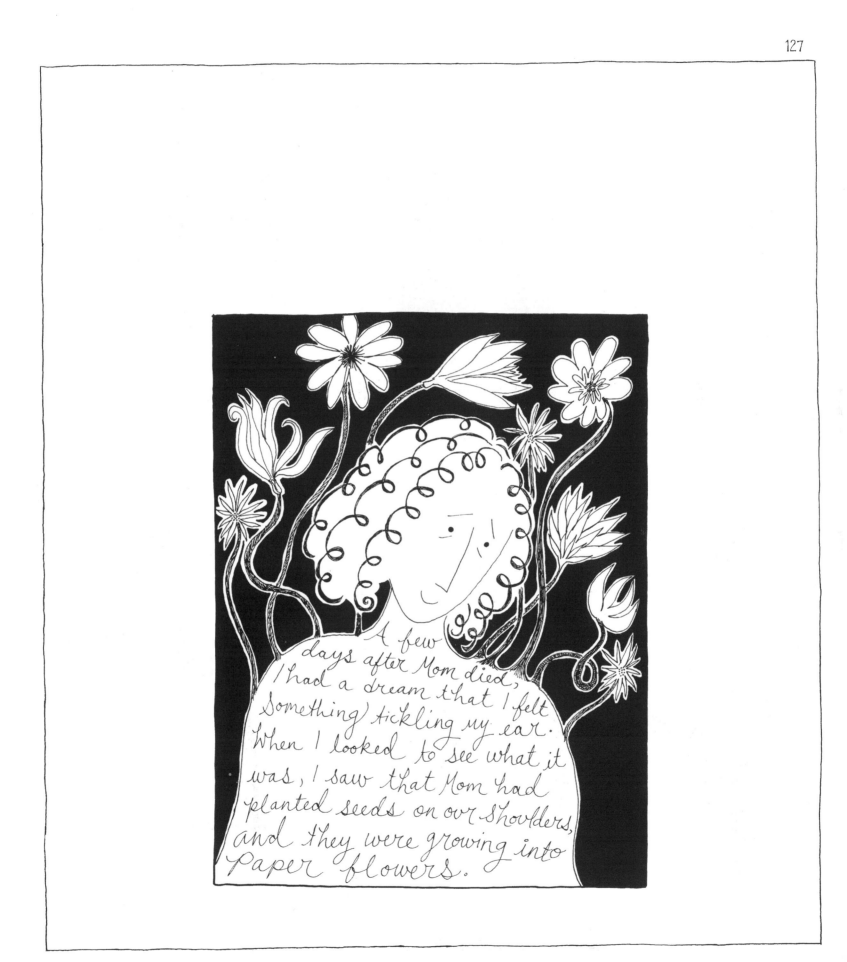

A few days after Mom died, I had a dream that I felt Something tickling my ear. When I looked to see what it was, I saw that Mom had planted seeds on our shoulders, and they were growing into Paper flowers.

Acknowledgements

I am overwhelmingly grateful to everyone who made this book a reality. Donimo was my rock, my link to sanity, my first reader, and my ass-kicker through the years of Mom's illness and the years of the writing process. My "drawing clinic" partner Mary Schendlinger kept me going with weekly drawing dates, constant encouragement, reality checks, and lots of food. My father Robert patiently and enthusiastically read my traumatic stories about his beloved Midge, and filled in some of the details about my mother's past (of course all errors are my own). Thanks to my agent Samantha Haywood for her excitement about the book, hard work, and determination; Robyn Read and Sarah Ivany at Freehand for their patience, support, and commitment; and the incredible Natalie Olsen of Kisscut Design for polishing my pages into a finished book. Last, but not least, I could not do anything without my wonderful friends, who encourage me, put up with my whining and periods of despair, share my joys, and create the incredible, sparkly, creative community where I live and work.

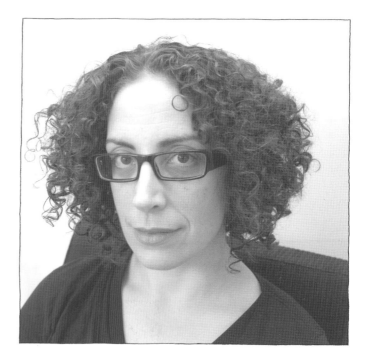

Sarah Leavitt writes both prose and comics. Her writing has appeared in Geist, The Globe and Mail, Vancouver Review, The Georgia Straight, and Xtra West. Leavitt has written short documentaries for Definitely Not the Opera on CBC Radio, and her non-fiction has appeared in a number of anthologies, including Nobody's Mother (Heritage 2006) and Beyond Forgetting: Poetry and Prose about Alzheimer's Disease (Kent State University Press 2009). She has an MFA in Creative Writing from UBC. Tangles is her first book.